Broadcast Pharmaceutical Advertising in the United States

Broadcast Pharmaceutical Advertising in the United States

Primetime Pill Pushers

Janelle Applequist, Ph.D.

LEXINGTON BOOKS
Lanham • Boulder • New York • London

Published by Lexington Books
An imprint of The Rowman & Littlefield Publishing Group, Inc.
4501 Forbes Boulevard, Suite 200, Lanham, Maryland 20706
www.rowman.com

Unit A, Whitacre Mews, 26–34 Stannary Street, London SE11 4AB

British Library Cataloguing in Publication Information Available

Library of Congress Cataloging-in-Publication Data
Names: Applequist, Janelle, author.
Title: Broadcast pharmaceutical advertising in the United States : primetime
  pill pushers / Janelle Applequist.
Description: Lanham : Lexington Books, [2016] | Includes bibliographical
  references and index.
Identifiers: LCCN 2016037293 (print) | LCCN 2016038340 (ebook) |
  ISBN 9781498539517 (cloth : alk. paper) | ISBN 9781498539524 (Electronic)
Subjects: | MESH: Pharmaceutical Preparations--economics | Direct-to-Consumer
  Advertising | Television--economics | United States
Classification: LCC HF6161.D7 (print) | LCC HF6161.D7 (ebook) |
  NLM QV 736 AA1 | DDC 659.19/61510973—dc23
LC record available at https://lccn.loc.gov/2016037293

Printed in the United States of America

For Shredder

Contents

List of Tables

Preface

Arguably, anyone who has watched television can immediately recognize that the phrase "ask your doctor about…" is associated with a pharmaceutical advertisement. When prompted, most can imagine at least one brand-name drug and describe its advertisement, whether it be the use of a couple in separate bath tubs signifying an ad for Cialis, a "purple pill" and its association with Nexium, or a celebrity testimonial testifying how a medication improved his or her life. Whether one can actually name what these drugs are meant to treat, the fact remains that brand association with pharmaceutical drugs in the United States is high, particularly in regard to the medium of broadcast television (Chandler and Owen 2002). Beyond informing consumers about pharmaceutical drugs on the market, these advertisements additionally model and promote prescription drug use as forms of consumer health interventions.

In recent decades, the role of patients in medical decision making has shifted. Patients are no longer viewed as passive recipients of health care information, but instead as active agents who play a key role in the medical decision-making processes (Frosch and Kaplan 1999). Being that pharmaceutical drugs are one of the few consumer products that require federal approval prior to entering commerce, it becomes all the more necessary that these products are advertised in a way that provides clear and truthful information, as these drugs have the potential to cause serious bodily harm. Beyond serving as informative of the health conditions these drugs are designed to treat, these advertisements serve as models for how lives can be improved by the use of medications. By using particular portrayals of characters and purposeful story lines that encourage consumption of these drugs, direct-to-consumer advertising (DTCA) sells the notion that these products offer additional benefits beyond one's health – essentially promising a happier life, more personal fulfillment, and even an increase in the quality of one's self-esteem

xi

and relationships. DTCA relies primarily on emotional appeals rather than utilizing informational or educational aspects, with most advertisements providing minimal health information, describing the benefits of taking a drug in vague, qualitative terms that rarely rely on scientific evidence to support the claims being made (Brownfield et al. 2004; Department of Health and Human Services 2010; Farris and Wilkie 2005; Fornell and Larcker 1981).

Pharmaceutical advertising is an area that merits debate, as the product available for consumption is one that can endanger the human body in a way that other advertised products cannot – in dealing with matters of health, consumer culture enters a realm that rests on the body and societal constructions of what it means to be "sick" and simultaneously what it means to be "healthy." DTCA is both a major source of information about drugs and health in the United States, and a major source of advertising funding for our media system. Profoundly contributing to the discourse and dynamics of U.S. health care, direct-to-consumer (DTC) advertisements alter the relationship between physicians and patients, by elevating pharmaceuticals as an important and necessary element for living the good life, ultimately reconfiguring how individuals perceive their own agency in this realm. Although the area has been extensively studied by health and media researchers, the scope of DTCA and the ways it may change over time makes it an ever-important area of study. Advertisements involve myriad elements for analysis, including visual imagery, sound, movement, and the list goes on. Therefore, beginning conversations about what messages these advertisements are conveying, how they may shape conversations one has with their health care provider, and implications for larger sociological understandings of health become all the more important.

From a research perspective, despite much solid content work on DTCA, arguably there are areas to still be explored. Two such limitations are emphases on print versions of DTC advertisements and a fairly circumscribed range of persuasive appeals in the ads. Think about a popular pharmaceutical advertisement. Chances are, you are envisioning and remembering a pharmaceutical advertisement you viewed on television, as this medium is the most popular for the industry. While emphases on print versions of pharmaceutical advertisements (e.g. in magazines) are certainly important, broadcast versions cannot be ignored, as this is the area that receives the most attention by media consumers. Another limitation of research focusing on the pharmaceutical industry's advertising efforts is the use of methodological approaches that are largely quantitative. Mixed-methods analyses are not common within this literature, most often utilizing either quantitative or qualitative approaches (Faerber and Kreling 2014; Frosch et al.2007; Gooblar and Carpenter 2013; Kaphingst et al. 2004; Yang et al. 2012). Quantitative research has a much larger presence (Faerber and Kreling 2014; Frosch et al. 2007; Kaphingst et al. 2004; Yang et al. 2012) and when qualitative frameworks are used, analyses are most often performed on a historical level, tracing the Food and Drug Administration (FDA)'s role in pharmaceutical advertising and presenting both sides of the "pharmaceutical advertising debate." Although highly important, few critical works on DTCA as presenting limited courses of health prevention have been published (Landau 2011; Quesinberry Stokes 2013). Again, while quantitative representations are vital in order to establish an empirical foundation for where we stand in relation to pharmaceutical advertising, richer, more descriptive analyses must also be introduced into the conversation. Take your own experience with health care, for example. Imagine visiting with your health care provider regarding recent bloodwork you had completed. Your physician provides you with a printout of your lab results (represented via numbers in a series of ranges and levels). Upon verbally telling you an issue found with a particular level of your bloodwork, the physician exits the room. Where is the explanation? Would your first thoughts not be to ask questions, to seek answers about the data with which you were just presented? This scenario is precisely why we must give lip service to asking more critical questions of an industry that so directly influences our health care.

Given the above limitations of research, dialogue, and debate – a narrow range of research questions dealing with factual claims and accuracy, a focus on print advertisements, and uni-dimensional approaches to methods – the goal of this book is to provide an empirical foundation regarding specific DTC advertisements in order to more critically and qualitatively analyze and discuss the content of these advertisements. In the case of DTCA, a mixed-methods approach is useful because quantitative content analysis can present a strong foundation (via findings) to paint a basic statistical picture regarding the current state of prescription drug advertisements, which can then be more deeply analyzed in order to discuss the implications associated with more critical concepts such as medicalization and pharmaceuticalization in the U.S. health care system, as shown through prominent examples and rich qualitative description. A more qualitative analysis can shed light on the implications for meaning-making these advertisements have for media consumers. By more descriptively presenting and discussing the content of these advertisements, the types of individuals being represented can better be explored. For example, are there significant patterns in terms of gender, race, socioeconomic status, etc. being shown? Furthermore, how are patients being portrayed? If individuals are shown as being active, healthy, and happy during the majority of these advertisements, then these traits are being sold alongside a product, influencing an individual's choice to speak with their doctor about beginning a medication regimen.

This book argues that the symbolic complexity of television DTC advertisements not only attempts to influence the drugs' perceived effectiveness, but also how drugs are used as key interventions in life, and portrayed to solve a host of personal and social problems. At the same time, the way that people are portrayed in DTCA also has implications for the mediated representations of gender, age, class and other social categories.

The following chapter provides an analysis of the prescription drug industry and common advertising strategies. Key moments in the history of DTCA regulation include the FDA's passing of the Kefauver-Harris Drug Amendment in 1962, giving the FDA authority over the release and marketing of prescription drugs and the FDA's Modernization Act in 1997, which deregulated the industry and relaxed restrictions necessary for prescription drug advertising. Additionally, chapter two will summarize the arguments made by proponents of the industry while addressing the negative associations often discussed in terms of patient safety. Finally, the chapter will discuss research on the effects of pharmaceutical advertising, finding that consumers recognize, associate with, and request these brands when visiting with their physicians.

The theoretical orientations of my arguments and the scholarship likely to be most influential will be detailed in chapter three, emphasizing a critical approach to DTCA. Critical Advertising Studies will be engaged and integrated throughout this book, which emphasizes two main areas of research: advertising as a cultural system and advertising as a funding system (McAllister and West 2013). Advertising as a cultural system involves looking at such issues as representation in advertising and how advertising offers a commodity as a solution to a social or personal problem (McAllister and West 2013). Examples of representation could include gender, race, class, able-bodiedness, and nationality, among others (Goffman 1979). In such cases, scholars address how advertising contributes to cultural constructions of social identity; such identities are embedded in power relations and are at their heart ideological.

Critical Advertising Studies is part of the larger paradigm of critical-cultural media studies. Critical approaches to culture were seen as early as the 1920s through work from the Frankfurt School, which by the 1930s included theorists Horkheimer, Adorno, Fromm, Marcuse, Lowenthal, and Benjamin (Kellner and Durham 2012). Such work began the critical tradition of exploring how media perpetuates or challenges social and cultural inequities. The Frankfurt School, strongly influenced by the works of Karl Marx and contextualized by the rise of both fascism and industrial capitalism, examined popular culture through the lens of media as a powerful creator, emphasizing the media's subsequent repression of other economic and cultural forces that could lead to social change and true progressive thought. One of the most influential essays by Horkheimer and Adorno, originally written in the 1940s (reprinted in 2002), focused on both the standardizing and narcotizing elements of mass culture, but also the entrenchment of advertising as a cultural form. Horkheimer and Adorno's *The Culture Industry: Enlightenment as Mass Deception* analyzes the mass industrialization imposed on cultural production as a totalizing system where culture is structured to benefit the larger cultural industry, and functions by disallowing the potential for human individuality, yet this piece repeatedly emphasizes that the existence of human individuality in modern industrialized culture is a myth (Horkheimer and Adorno 1972). Rather, the culture industry promotes forms of pseudo-individuality in which trivial differences are falsely offered as genuine options for life decisions, therefore co-opting true individuality. Related to this understanding of individuality is Foucault's philosophy on defining power or uniqueness in terms of its ability to take action. That is, individuals are not linear, passive creatures, but rather, active beings whose actions inevitably overlap with the actions of others, thereby making it impossible to consider an individual without also taking into account the context of their social presence (Foucault 1983).

Critical Advertising Studies will be described in addition to outlining how the processes of medicalization, pharmaceuticalization, and commodity fetishism are useful in describing consumerist orientations present in prescription drug marketing. Traditional views on medicalization come from the field of sociology and approach the construction of disease, highlighting how medical expansion has permitted an increased sense of control over the lives of individuals and an expanded definition of what is "illness" (Williams, Gabe, and Davis 2008). While the utilization of the theory of medicalization is important in order to describe sociological constructions of health, it is my intent to offer a mass communications/media studies approach that can focus more on the constructions of health, patients, and pharmaceutical drugs via media platforms. More traditional health communication has positioned medicine as a form of cultural authority that is apolitical, meaning its only existence is to improve the health of citizens (McAllister 1992). Medicalization is an attempt to deconstruct these notions, as it highlights how medical ideology has intersected into our everyday lives, often allowing the "difficulties people have" to be transformed into illness, disease, or instances that require professional medical intervention (McAllister 1992; Engelhardt 1986). Media discourses about health and medicine can serve, then, as a source for or against medicalized definitions. Chapter three will also introduce the concept of "pharmaceutical fetishism," the foundation for this book, arguing that this is a useful term for the analysis of DTCA and its conceptions of health care and patient representation.

Chapter four extends upon previous DTCA research by conducting a quantitative content analysis (providing an empirical foundation) of 805 broadcast prescription drug advertisements from 2010 (featuring 36 unique advertisements for 25 different prescription drugs), with coding categories

accounting for previously used approaches to DTCA emphasizing categories of informational and/or educational content. This chapter addresses the
educational and/or informational aspects of DTCA. The chapter concludes
that DTC advertisements undermine their informational function by emphasizing overwhelmingly positive outcomes of drug use and discouraging serious considerations of risk factors and other treatment options.

Chapter five provides a more detailed and nuanced interpretation of critical
variables to be considered in DTCA, discussing important themes found in
the empirical sample utilized and the ways in which these themes fit in with
the previously mentioned concepts of medicalization, pharmaceuticalization,
and most importantly, pharmaceutical fetishism. The chapter analyzes important issues of patient representation via grounded theory and textual analyses.
The goal of this chapter is to critically evaluate and understand pharmaceutical advertisements as commercial and ideological texts, in order to more fully
understand the degree to which these promotional forms reinforce or perhaps
question social trends of commercialized health care. The majority of DTCA
research has emphasized its use of emotional appeals and increased cases of
prescribing by doctors. This book more directly interprets the meanings of
the most popular ads themselves by outlining the ways in which the pharmaceutical industry frames conceptions of health in the United States. This book
explains how pharmaceutical advertisements are explicitly utilizing the
"magic" of advertising by presenting prescription drugs as cures for more
than just health conditions. Drugs are advertised in a way that presents them
as having the added benefit of selling a particular lifestyle to individuals – one
that emphasizes happiness, successful relationships, nuclear family activities, and personal fulfillment. Furthermore, these ads perpetuate normalized
conceptions of particular representations, featuring characters that portray
stereotypical gender roles, youthfulness even in cases of being older, heteronormative relationships, familial relationships as being central to health, and
patients as being autonomous from their physicians. This means that drugs
have been commodified to sell much more than remedies for health conditions. Commodity fetishism is the relationship between people and products,
and fetishism occurs once individuals see meaning in things that seem an
inherent part of their physical existence, yet, the meaning is actually created
by individuals themselves (Marx 1992). Thus, products appear to have value
inherent in them, but the fact is that human beings themselves produce the
additional value. Advertisements allow for culture to associate products with
meaning, as emotional meaning, forms of promotional culture, and even
logos and branding animation (i.e. the use of animation in pharmaceutical
advertisements) can evoke sentiment for individuals (Williams 1980).

Chapter six presents content and textual analyses of one prescription drug
advertisement rospirenone/ethinyl estradiol (YAZ) in an effort to demonstrate

how DTCA circumvents the process of the doctor-patient relationship, ultimately allowing the patient to feel they have a sense of autonomy or authority. The concept of pharmaceutical fetishism relies upon the forms of pseudo-autonomy presented to consumers, namely through DTC advertisements. The YAZ advertisement analyzed in this chapter serves as an example of the ways in which the pharmaceutical industry celebrates the commodity that is the prescription drug, simultaneously giving less service to the potential harm associated with consumption of these products. By continuously reaffirming the positive aspects associated with YAZ, Bayer Pharmaceuticals has performed a type of pharmaceutical fetishism that presents the oral contraceptive as having the ability to deliver much more than its intended uses. The context provided offers an important look at the multiple platforms used by prescription drug industry in its marketing of health and products available for consumption. In particular, the chapter emphasizes gendered portrayals seen throughout a specific campaign and its consumption-oriented messages and the ways in which these concepts relate to instances of disease branding/disease mongering.

The final chapter concludes by offering a discussion of the text overall, providing an overview of the major themes apparent in pharmaceutical advertising, implications for society, and considerations for moving forward to protect consumers from misinformation associated with their health care.

Acknowledgments

First and foremost, I offer my sincerest gratitude to Dr. Michael Elavsky, who has supported me throughout my undergraduate, masters, and doctoral programs with his insight, support, and knowledge while allowing me to have the room to develop into the scholar I have become. I am also indebted to his family: Steriani, Misha, Ellie, and Natalka, who have each become such a special part of my life. I also equally attribute the meaning of my doctoral degree to Dr. Matthew P. McAllister, as his encouragement and positive example, both in and out of the classroom, have remained constant throughout my graduate career. As my co-advisers and co-chairs, Dr. Elavsky and Dr. McAllister have made it truly an honor to be their advisee, as they have each instilled in me that it is possible to make a difference. A graduate student simply could not wish for better sources of knowledge, guidance, and mentorship, and I hope to someday pay that forward with my students.

Dr. Fuyuan Shen and Dr. Jon Nussbaum have been invaluable to me not only while writing this dissertation, but also in the classroom. Each taught me the importance of approaching research in a way that allows all angles to be explored, and they taught me to do so with integrity. For that, I will always be grateful. It has truly been a pleasure to work with my committee.

This page would not be complete without expressing my thanks and love to my graduate student colleagues, who made my experience in graduate school as memorable as it was. Finally, to my parents and my brothers, thank you for instilling the values in me that promote my drive and determination while reminding me to enjoy life as I continue my journey. Without each of you, I could not have made it this far. And, of course, I cannot forget Shredder, my favorite puppy to come home to every night after a long day of researching, teaching, and writing.

Chapter 1

The Nature of the Pharmaceutical Advertising Industry

Direct-to-Consumer Advertising in the United States

Direct-to-consumer advertising (DTCA) is defined as any paid form of mediated communication for prescription drugs, the effect of which is to "induce the prescription, supply, purchase, and/or use of those (prescription) medicines" (Kotler and Keller 2006). Forms of DTC publicity can include, but are not limited to, radio commercials, magazine advertisements, television commercials, and Internet banner ads or pop-ups. The United States and New Zealand are the only two countries in the world that legally permit the direct advertisement of prescription drugs to consumers. In fact, as will be argued, in the United States DTCA is a major category of advertisements featured in media. It is important to recognize the ways in which these advertisements are regulated and enacted because their heavy presence in the media have the possibility of impacting serious and personal health care choices that individuals make with their physicians.

DTCA in the United States has become one of the most influential sectors in terms of its profit-making ability and its impact on consumer decisions. No longer relying solely on physicians to suggest medications, the pharmaceutical industry continues to invest in the advertising sector to influence what is undeniably a profitable industry: the pharmaceutical consumer. The pervasiveness of DTCA may influence patient perceptions of care, as Americans spend a mean of approximately 15 minutes per year with a doctor, yet spend more than 16 hours a year viewing DTCA on television (Brownfield et al. 2004). According to the Centers for Disease Control and Prevention, in 2013, about half of all Americans took at least one prescription drug per month, with 10% taking more than four (U.S. Department of Health 2014). In that year, Americans spent more than $263 billion on prescription drugs, accounting for 9.7% of all national health expenditures (U.S. Department of Health 2014). The pharmaceutical industry spent $4.34 billion on United States DTCA in 2010, increasing more than four times the $0.70 billion spent in

1996 (Kantar Media 2011). During a time when most industries seem to be struggling to survive in the turbulent economy, the pharmaceutical industry seems to be unaffected. The profit motive of the pharmaceutical industry is clear, as research suggests that for every $1.00 spent on pharmaceutical advertising, pharmaceutical retail sales increase by $4.20, with this amount increasing each year (Rosenthal et al. 2003).

Such pervasive economic and cultural dynamics are not neutral. As will be discussed, with the ubiquity of DTCA, the brand-name drug sector is given precedence over the generic sector, mainly through interconnected corporate and government relationships that provide the pharmaceutical sector with access to the agencies that yield the greatest amounts of power. In addition, an emphasis on pharmaceutical solutions to health concerns is highlighted in DTCA. DTCA also may be characterized by specific textual characteristics that position health and human agency in particular ways that accentuate their pervasiveness. There may be definite patterns to DTCA that present issues of life, health, health care, and drug use as non-neutral and with definitive ideological and cultural implications.

THE HISTORICAL EVOLUTION OF DRUG ADVERTISING

The first DTC advertisements to exist featured those for patent medicines in American newspapers in 1708. Patent medicines were advertised for the next 200 years through newspapers, magazines, and traveling medicine shows. Beginning in the early 1800s, the media and pharmaceutical industry had created a dependent relationship, with newspapers receiving their highest income from advertising, and patient medicine advertisers being willing to spend more on advertising than any other industry (Young 1969). The first federal legislation requiring complete labeling of dosage instructions and ingredients for medications was not passed until 1906. This was the Pure Food and Drugs Act, also known as the Wiley Act, and was put in place to ensure that individuals could clearly read and understand all drug labels (The Pure Food and Drugs Act 1906). The Wiley Act required that information on drug labels could only contain descriptions relevant to the drug's actual uses, meaning that it could not claim uses for which it was not originally created, and a drug was also required to list all ingredients. While this legislation helped to ensure that patients had the opportunity to read and understand what medication(s) they were consuming, it surprisingly did not require that any drugs be deemed safe for human use prior to marketing (The Pure Food and Drugs Act 1906). Essentially, this meant that medications remained on the market, even if they were physically harmful for consumers, as long as product labeling was present.

It is important to contextualize the effects of the 1906 Wiley Act. Food, drug, and cosmetics advertising increased significantly in magazines, newspapers, and radio following the act. As Congress began to see an increase in these types of advertisements, they began to understand the importance of protecting consumers from fraudulent marketing (i.e. product advertisements making untruthful claims) (The Pure Food and Drugs Act 1906). For this reason, in 1938, the Federal Food, Drug, and Cosmetic Act (FDCA) was passed. The FDCA required that all medications be proven safe prior to marketing efforts (Gellad and Lyles 2007). This act is also significant because it established the FDA. Congress gave the FDA authority to regulate the labeling of all drugs, but the Federal Trade Commission (FTC) had authority over all drug advertising (The Federal Food, Drug, and Cosmetic Act 1938).

DEVELOPMENT OF DIRECT-TO-CONSUMER REGULATION

Prior to 1951, the only medications given by a doctor that by law required a prescription were narcotics. As concerns over DTCA grew with the increased presence of print and radio advertisements for over-the-counter (OTC) medications, Congress recognized that prescription drugs needed to be regulated more closely in order to protect the public. In 1951, the Durham-Humphrey Amendments to the FDCA were passed, requiring that drugs deemed safe only for use under the care of a medical doctor be dispensed through a written prescription from that licensed practitioner (Durham-Humphrey Amendments 1951). It was at this time that advertisers began to see physicians as a target market for the prescription drug market, meaning that OTC medications were no longer the only opportunity for advertising health care treatment options.

In 1954, the FTC and FDA reached a working agreement in order to avoid any duplicate efforts being made to protect the public. Instead of the FDA having jurisdiction over all drug labeling, and the FTC having authority over all advertising, conversations between the two regulatory agencies began in order to devise a way to best serve the public. In 1962, the Kefauver-Harris Drug Amendment to the FDCA gave all regulatory authority of drug advertising from the FTC to the FDA (United States Kefauver-Harris Amendment 1962). This transfer of authority came largely in part as a result of the thalidomide tragedy, when thalidomide treatments used to treat nausea in pregnant women were not tested for toxicity, causing severe birth defects in thousands of infants (Kim and Scialli 2011). It is interesting to note that, at that time, DTC advertisements for prescription drugs did not have a strong presence for the general public, but were beginning to be seen in print formats directed toward physicians who were now seen as having more cultural authority in their ability to prescribe drugs for patients. OTC medications were what were heavily advertised to consumers, meaning that, at that time, the amendment never specifically addressed whether the FDA had control over prescription drug advertising. Congress was mainly concerned with advertisements directed toward the medical community because they were seen as the gatekeepers in terms of prescribing drugs (Calfee 2002). The FDCA was amended again in 1968 to reflect the increasing presence of DTC advertisements in print format, giving the FDA explicit and primary authority over prescription drug advertising. Additionally, this amendment allowed the FDA to provide explicit guidelines for prescription drug advertising (Palumbo and Mullins 2002).

After the FDA was given jurisdiction over DTCA in 1968, the agency required all drug companies to provide a "brief summary requirement" for all medications advertised to physicians, and at that time, it only applied to print advertisements because broadcast advertisements had not yet come to fruition. The "brief summary requirement" essentially meant that, in print advertisements, drug companies had to provide a summary of the product, including any risk-related information, with all promotional material (Food and Drug Administration Modernization Act 1997). The FDA defines the "brief summary" in one paragraph, stating: "Advertisements must disclose each side effect, warning, precaution, and contraindication from the approved product professional labeling. FDA-approved patient labeling that focuses on the most serious risks and less serious, but most frequently occurring, adverse reactions is also acceptable." ("FDA's division of" 2004). Therefore, any print advertisements under the "brief summary requirement" had to include all warnings, major precautions, and the three to five most common "non-serious adverse reactions most likely to affect the patient's quality of life in compliance with drug therapy" (Gellad and Lyles 2007).

Through the 1970s, pharmaceutical companies focused their promotional efforts on physicians because the language involved in providing the "brief summary" was seen as too convoluted for patients to understand. Additionally, it seemed to be too much of a challenge for pharmaceutical companies to disclose all of the potential side effects to the public while still making their product seem appealing. It was not until 1981 that the pharmaceutical industry proposed changes in its marketing efforts to include consumers, citing the "educational" benefit of pharmaceutical advertising as a source of public knowledge (Wilkes, Bell, and Kravitz 2000). Simultaneously, political and regulatory climates, which were centered on deregulation and a greater level of lenience toward the pharmaceutical industry's business initiatives, were moving toward allowing consumers to have greater choices, offering patients more opportunity to be "empowered" in their medical decision making (Shuchman and Wilkes 1994). Social deterministic approaches began to serve as underpinnings for conceptions of health, growing largely since the 1950s with Paolo Friere's work which shed light on an oppressor-oppressed relationship in society, with this framework extending through the civil rights movement in the 1960s, and finally coming to fruition as a result of the self-help movement seen in the 1980s, centering patient empowerment as a form of self-management, productivity, and human agency (Chambers and Thompson 2008; Finfgeld 2004; Laverack 2009; Pulvirenti, McMillan, and Lawn 2011). Beginning in 1981, the FDA required that print advertisements, now directed at consumers, be held to the same standards as the "brief summary requirement" put in place for marketing tactics aimed at physicians. This decision limited the presence of print DTC advertisements in the 1980s because pharmaceutical companies still felt that the "brief summary requirement" would make consumers more fearful about taking a medication. Being required to list all of the potential side effects often times takes up three to four pages in a magazine advertisement, and this can understandably seem frightening for a consumer, therefore negating the original intent of the advertisement itself (Lyles 2002).

SIGNIFICANT POLICY CHANGES FOR DTC BROADCAST ADVERTISEMENTS: THE MODERNIZATION ACT OF 1997

Prior to 1997, DTC advertisements were seen in print formats, directed at physicians and consumers. Yet, their popularity did not take off exponentially until the FDA significantly amended DTC advertisement guidelines in 1997. Beginning in 1995, the FDA held public hearings for pharmaceutical companies to speak about DTC promotional efforts. Two years later, in 1997, the FDA issued a report concerning the manufacturer dissemination of advertisements for prescription drugs specifically associated with broadcast media. This was the first time the FDA acknowledged the ability of prescription drug manufacturers to have their advertisements seen on television (Palumbo and Mullins 2002). In 1997, the final guidelines were released by the FDA, permitting prescription drug advertisements to be seen by consumers on television, as long as advertisers fulfilled the requirements put in place. This was the FDA's Modernization Act of 1997 (Food and Drug Administration Modernization Act 1997).

One of the main arguments posited by pharmaceutical companies during the public hearings was that the "brief summary requirement" was unfair because thirty-second commercials on television could not possibly list all of the side effects and potential risk factors in such a limited amount of time. The FDA responded by amending the "brief summary requirement" for broadcast advertisements only to become the "adequate provision requirement."

The FDA explains that "...in place of the brief summary, advertisements may make 'adequate provision' for dissemination of package labeling with four alternative sources of information: a toll-free telephone number, a referral to a print advertisement in a concurrently running print publication, a referral to a health care provider, or an Internet web page address" (Food and Drug Administration Modernization Act 1997). This is why every broadcast DTC advertisement explicitly states for consumers to "ask their doctor about...," "see our ad in (magazine)," or to "visit this website for more information." Instead of broadcast prescription drug advertisers providing all of the risk information during a commercial, they directed consumers to alternative sources for finding that information on their own. The advertisements are required to fulfill the "major statement," meaning that information must be included about the major risks of a drug and only the most common side effects (Food and Drug Administration Modernization Act 1997). This practice is dangerous and highly problematic, as it permits pharmaceutical companies, not the FDA, to have the power to deem what is "most serious" or "most significant" in the lives of consumers.

Once these guidelines were finalized and introduced by 1999, DTCA on television was born, and became standard industry practice. Top pharmaceutical companies spend more money every year (approximately $160 million) on broadcast advertising than other well-known consumer goods, including Budweiser ($146 million), Pepsi ($125 million), and Nike ($78 million) (United States Government Accountability Office 2006). The influence of this industry extends beyond advertising and to the interconnected relationships that exist with the very agency put in place to protect consumer safety.

MAJOR PLAYERS IN THE BRAND-NAME PHARMACEUTICAL SECTOR: A POWER STRUCTURE ANALYSIS

Pharmaceutical industry lobbyists are main actors in the health care industry. Since 1998, the pharmaceutical industry has remained the largest spender on lobbying in the United States, spending over $225 million in 2013 alone (U.S. Senate 2014). In 2013, over 1400 drug-industry lobbyists worked in Washington, versus 100 senators and 435 representatives, making the drug industry represented nearly three times that of elected members of Congress in Washington, D.C. (U.S. Senate 2014).

Brand-name drug manufacturers generate more revenue to the federal government than generic companies, making their influence with lawmakers in Washington much greater. This revenue comes in the form of industry user fees, which generates half of the budget for the FDA. According to the FDA:

Under sections 735 and 736 of the Federal Food, Drug, and Cosmetic Act (21 U.S.C. 379g and 379h), the FDA has the authority to assess and collect user fees for certain drug and biologics license applications and supplements. Under this authority, pharmaceutical companies pay fees for certain new human drug applications, biologics applications, and supplements submitted to the agency for review (Kenneth and DiMassi 2000).

Beginning in 1992, the Prescription Drug User Fees Act made the FDA dependent on funding from pharmaceutical firms, creating a form of regulatory capture. As the FDA relied more on funding from the pharmaceutical industry, the industry began to demand more rapid reviews of applications for new drugs, which researchers have claimed resulted in an "epidemic of insufficiently-tested drugs" (Light, Lexchin, and Darrow 2013). Brand-name drug manufacturers pay higher industry user fees to the FDA, which means that the more expensive a drug, the higher the fee a manufacturer pays. The FDA then receives the most money in industry user fees from those medications that are brand names and have the highest price tags for consumers. Essentially, it is most financially beneficial for the FDA when brand-name drugs get approved. It is not surprising then that multiple members of advisory committees for the FDA have direct business ties to these brand-name industries, either through employment or stock ownership (Kenneth and DiMassi 2000). These advisory committees are the groups that make the final recommendations on drug approval, suggesting that brand-name drug companies have greater power over the generic drug sector. The phenomenon of the revolving door, the flow of high-ranking industry personnel into the government regulatory sector, has been a common practice for the FDA, exemplifying a type of institutional corruption that permits the pharmaceutical industry to exert its influence in government affairs, compromising the very legislation meant to protect the public from unsafe drugs (Meghani and Kuzma 2011). In perhaps the best example of the pharmaceutical industry's revolving door, in 2004, Representative Billy Tauzin of Louisiana retired as chairman of the House committee that regulated the pharmaceutical industry to become the president and CEO of the drug industry's top lobbying group, the Pharmaceutical Research and Manufacturers of America (PhRMA) (Welch 2004). PhRMA is one of the most powerful lobbying firms in Washington, having led the lobbying efforts that successfully passed a bill overhauling Medicare. Receiving a pay package of more than $2 million a year, Tauzin became one of the highest paid lobbyists in Washington.

The interconnected ties of ownership in the pharmaceutical industry extend beyond the FDA and also directly raise the issue of media and bank ownership and control. The pharmaceutical industry is heavily positioned via representation on the boards of directors of media corporations. As Matt Carlson (2001) wrote, "the chair and CEO of Eli Lilly sits on the board of Knight Ridder, the chair of Pfizer is on the board of Dow Jones, and the chair emeritus of Bristol-Myers Squibb and the president of Schering-Plough are both directors for the New York Times company" (Carlson 2001, 18). This leaves the media in a position of potential bias; creating an incentive for positive news coverage of brand-name drugs, while giving generic medication options little to no attention, or even negative claims. When a CEO has direct ties to an industry, their interests in that specific industry inevitably trickle down to owned and controlled television broadcast stations, thereby impacting not only the way in which stories are framed, but how often (if at all) they are made available to the public.

The brand-name pharmaceutical industry is made up of giant corporations. This industry is highly concentrated, demonstrating the nature of capitalism. Thirteen brand-name pharmaceutical companies made the "Fortune 500" list in 2013, with four of these companies placing in the top 100. Johnson & Johnson (ranked 41 with $67.2 billion in revenue), Pfizer (ranked 48 with $61.2 billion in revenue), Merck (ranked 58 with $47.3 billion in revenue), and Abbott Laboratories (ranked 70 with $39.9 billion in revenue) are viewed as the most influential leaders in the pharmaceutical industry ("Fortune 500: 2012" 2013). Seeing that the pharmaceutical industry has such a strong position in the market, its top players would rather control the market than actually compete. Hence, the pharmaceutical economy is oligopolistic.

The U.S. economy has a dual structure, comprised of core companies (those on the Fortune 500 list), and the roughly 23 million mid-sized or small businesses located on the periphery (Bowles and Edwards 1993). Core firms have substantial market power, whereas periphery firms have little market power. Bowles and Edwards wrote that the goal of giant corporations, such as those in the pharmaceutical industry, is to exist within a shared monopoly that has unwritten rules for business. Each corporation accepts the unwritten rules because it is more profitable to abide by the rules than to violate them (Bowles and Edwards 1993). The first rule these corporations follow is to avoid price competition. In doing so, more cooperative pricing efforts result, meaning that four or five major firms still have all the opportunity (Bowles and Edwards 1993). A second major rule that is followed is to create "new products." The advantage to a corporation having more items to advertise is that consumers will be more likely to notice that corporation's products – they are exposed to that corporation more often. The pharmaceutical industry is successful at making consumers become more aware of their products, introducing new drugs to the market multiple times a year. Although it seems as if new prescription drugs are constantly being introduced to potential patients via their television screens each year, multiple independent reviews have concluded that 85–90% of drugs introduced to the public over the last 15 years have provided "few or no clinical advantages for patients" (Angell 2004; Hunt 2000; Morgan et al. 2005; Motola et al. 2006; van Luijn et al. 2010).

Finally, top pharmaceutical companies focus on increasing their shares as opposed to emphasizing price competition with other firms. To increase their market share, each corporation intensifies their sales efforts, including forms of advertising, marketing, and sales representation (Bowles and Edwards 1993). Beyond corporate decisions made in the boardroom, pharmaceutical sales representatives, in particular, serve as intermediaries for the prescription drug industry, often becoming part of the ideological process that positions pills as commodities in the sense that these representatives genuinely believe they are promulgating a positive process for health care. One of the most influential pieces of literature regarding the training practices for pharmaceutical sales representatives is a result of litigation between the Attorney General Prescriber/Consumer Education Program and Warner-Lambert, a division of Pfizer. Claiming that consumer protection laws were being violated by marketing campaigns for the drug Neurontin, a settlement was reached in 2004, which required that the hearing transcripts be made public in order to give consumers the ability to learn more about the violations of consumer protection laws by the prescription drug industry (Fugh-Berman and Ahari 2007). The released data includes insight from Shahram Ahari, a former drug representative for Eli Lilly, and Adriane Fugh-Berman, a physician who researches pharmaceutical marketing. As described, the relationship between a representative and a physician is based on acquisition and reciprocity. Ahari, having been an actor in the process, offers an exclusive perspective on the dynamic, saying, "It's my job to figure out what a physician's price is. For some, it's dinner at the finest restaurants, for others it's enough convincing data to let them prescribe confidently, and for others it's my attention and friendship…but at the most basic level, everything is for sale and everything is an exchange" (Fugh-Berman and Ahari 2007). Ahari often uses the term "friendship" in order to describe the network – it is never referred to as a business relationship, but rather, the approach taken is to befriend the physician. Sales representatives get their jobs based on their confidence, personality, and people skills. In return, they are expected to study the personalities, interests, and prescribing habits of medical professionals. By intimately getting to know their target, sales representatives build rapport with physicians, allowing each party to approach any exchanges from a friendly, comfortable angle.

Pharmaceutical sales representatives are trained extensively prior to going out in the field. Because successful detailing increases revenue, pharmaceutical companies do not cut costs when it comes to molding a future employee. The average cost to recruit, hire, and train a pharmaceutical sales representative is $89,000 (Goldberg and Davenport 2005). The primary aspect of training involves encouraging sales representatives to remember small details about specific physicians, which many scholars have suggested is the reason why sales representatives refer to their visits with physicians as "detailing." Representatives are taught to scan the offices of physicians, looking for family photos, alumni memorabilia, sporting equipment, or any other objects that can be used to establish personal and lasting connections (Fugh-Berman and Ahari 2007). This friendship becomes an association based on business exchanges, but one that is framed as being a meaningful, loyal kinship.

Research from the Kaiser Family Foundation has shown that out of 2,068 practicing physicians surveyed, three quarters found medical data provided by pharmaceutical drug representatives as "somewhat useful" (59%) or "very useful" (15%); yet, only 9% of physicians surveyed viewed this information as "very accurate," 72% felt it was "somewhat accurate," and 14% declared the data was "not very" or "not at all" accurate ("National Survey of Physicians" 2006). The relationship formed calls attention to the reliability of any information or data obtained. By viewing their source of information as a likeable companion, physicians may not be able to accurately identify when certain data is questionable or not medically sound. The ideological constructs of the physician and the sales representative become aligned as a result of the reciprocal association present. Once a sales representative establishes a connection, behaviors by the physician are rewarded. Pharmaceutical sales representatives strategically use gifting as an incentive system for prescribing medications. What is most interesting about this practice may not be its exclusivity, but its hierarchy in terms of handouts. The best, most expensive gifts are given to those physicians that prescribe at the highest rate. Essentially, the more a physician prescribes a certain medication, the greater return they see through an increase in the monetary value of the gifts given. Michael Oldani, a former pharmaceutical sales representative and anthropologist, has written that this system is carefully maintained with the core of pharmaceutical gifting being that, "bribes aren't considered bribes" (Elliott 2006).

Prescription tracking refers to the collection of big data in an effort to identify the highest-selling prescriptions. Information distribution companies (IMS Health, Dendrite, Verispan, Wolters Kluwer, etc.) purchase records from pharmacies. What many consumers do not realize is that most pharmacies have these records for sale, and are able to do so legally by not including patient names and only providing a physician's state licensing number (Steinbrook 2006). Yet, sales representatives are able to identify specific physicians through licensing agreements in place by the American Medical Association. The number-one customer for information distribution companies is the pharmaceutical industry, which purchases the prescribing data to identify the highest prescribers and also to track the effects of their promotional efforts. Physicians are given a "value," a ranking from one to ten, which identifies how often they prescribe drugs. A sales training guide for Merck even states that this value is, "used to identify which products are currently in favor with the physician in order to develop a strategy to change those prescriptions into Merck prescriptions" (Merck 2002). The empirical evidence provided by information distribution companies offers a glimpse into the personality, behaviors, and beliefs of a physician, which is why these numbers are so valued by the drug industry. Ron Brand, an employee of IMS, wrote, "integrated segmentation analyzes individual prescribing behaviors, demographics, and psychographics (attitudes, beliefs, and values) to fine-tune sales targets. For a particular product, for example, one segment might consist of price-sensitive physicians, another might include doctors loyal to a given manufacturers brand, and a third may include those unfriendly towards reps" (Brand and Kumar 2003). The prominence of the pharmaceutical industry's sales efforts can be seen through its investment in marketing and DTC advertisements, and the fact that this spending is greater than what is put toward research and development phases for diseases and cures.

While brand-name drug companies have continued to claim that higher medication prices are put in place to finance further research for new developments in health care remedies, data shows that advertising has taken precedence over experimentation for new treatment options. In 2012, the pharmaceutical industry spent more than $27 billion on drug promotion, comprised of $24 billion toward marketing to physicians via sales representatives and over $3 billion on advertising to consumers (mainly through television commercials) (Cegedim strategic data 2013). Conversely, that same year pharmaceutical manufacturers spent $1.9 billion on research and development (R&D) – this means that for every dollar pharmaceutical companies spent on research, $19 was spent on promotion and marketing efforts, outlining a clear imbalance between innovation and advertising (Light and Lexchin 2012). While brand-name drug companies have continued to claim that higher medication prices are put in place to finance further research for new developments, data suggests that advertising has taken precedence over experimentation, especially after the FDA's Modernization Act was passed in 1997. The United States Government Accountability Office reported that, from 1997 to 2001, of the nine top drug companies, DTC drug advertising and marketing costs increased 145%, while spending on research and development increased only 59% (United States Government Accountability Office 2002).

PROCESSES AND PRACTICES OF THE
BRAND-NAME DRUG INDUSTRY: "ME-TOO" DRUGS

Once the FDA approves a drug, it is given a brand-name patent that can last up to 20 years. This gives exclusivity to the manufacturer of the drug, allowing it an extended period of time where it is the only entity manufacturing and marketing the drug. It is only after the 20-year period that other manufacturers are permitted to have access to the drug's bio molecular formula in order to create a generic version. Not surprisingly, companies invest great amounts of money in marketing their medications during the first 20 years because this is the time when most of the profits are made (Rhee 2008).

One of the biggest problems that pharmaceutical companies face is patent expiration. Once the exclusivity rights for a drug expire, generic versions can enter the market, potentially putting a significant dent in the drug's profits. The development of the "me-too" drug has helped to counteract this problem. Me-too drugs enter the market most often when patents are soon set to expire, and are minor biomolecular variations of an already profitable drug. Pharmaceutical trade publications describe me-too drugs as a way to "extend the monopoly rights on an older blockbuster" (Marcia 2004). The pharmaceutical market is increasingly using me-too drugs, primarily because the target market and advertising tactics have already been established, meaning that this approach is cost-effective and less labor-intensive (Marcia 2004). From 1998 to 2003, the FDA approved 487 drugs. Of those, 379 (78%) were classified by the FDA as "appearing to have therapeutic qualities similar to those of one or more already marketed drugs, with 333 (68%) not even being new compounds, but instead being new formulations of combinations of old ones. Only 67 (14%) of the 487 were actually new compounds considered likely to be improvements over older drugs" (U.S. Food and Drug Administration 2004).

Nexium is a helpful example for describing the ways in which the pharmaceutical industry re-distributes a drug in order to retain exclusivity in the marketplace. During the late 1990s, Prilosec, a DTC-sold drug for gastrointestinal discomfort, was the number one selling drug in the world (Bernard and Wells 2015). Prilosec's corporation, AstraZeneca, introduced Nexium in the fall of 2001 when the patent for Prilosec was about to expire. In order to market Nexium, AstraZeneca had its scientists isolate an active ingredient in its prescription-only Prilosec, months before Prilosec was approved by the FDA to become available to patients as an OTC medication (not needing a prescription). This resulted in simultaneously creating a new molecule, esomeprazole. AstraZeneca was then able to get a new patent because of the added molecule, giving the corporation the entry point it needed in order to remain strong in the market (Bernard and Wells 2015). Rather than simply taking all of the advertising techniques directly from Prilosec, AstraZeneca developed a campaign to construct the "new and updated" drug as better than Prilosec. In order to be able to sell consumers this message, AstraZeneca designed its clinical trials to highlight two specific areas of improvement seen with Nexium versus Prilosec: acid reflux disease and stomach acid damage to the esophagus (Bernard and Wells 2015). Framing their clinical trials in this way opened the door for AstraZeneca to market Nexium as not only being better than Prilosec, but as being the best acid reflux product on the market. It was at this point, in 2001, that AstraZeneca sent its sales team out with published evidence that Nexium was superior.

Saatchi & Saatchi Healthcare Communications picked up AstraZeneca during this time and received the account for Nexium's marketing. According to pharmaceutical trade publications, Dave Marek, managing director for the account, had this to say regarding the agency's approach to advertising Nexium to consumers:

> We can take a message and just hit them [consumers] over the head with it time after time, but people tire of that very quickly. What's more meaningful is when they engage with the brand continuously, and have the ability to adjust the content to what's most important and relevant to them. We're putting a lot of effort into telling stories. People remember stories. They don't remember the facts. So encapsulating everything in the context of a story is a much more rich communication strategy that will stick in a customer's mind (Arnold 2009, 153).

Nexium has been described by the pharmaceutical industry as the most successful me-too drug in history. Only two years after entering the market, Nexium was the most highly advertised drug of 2004. The advertising budget for Nexium was $219 million, with $104 million of these costs going toward television advertising. In that same year, Nexium resulted in $3.3 billion in sales, and was ranked as the world's seventh-largest prescription drug (Bittar 2004). AstraZeneca's success in making Nexium a blockbuster drug with only two years of planning has been described as the most powerful example of marketing efforts in pharmaceutical history (Bittar 2004). In May of 2014, Nexium was launched as an OTC medication, no longer requiring a prescription. Generic versions of the former prescription-only drug have not yet reached the market due to a Consent Decree issued by the FDA concerning manufacturing violations, limiting the ability of imported pharmaceutical ingredients for the medication to the United States (McCaffrey 2014). This means that OTC Nexium may in fact be given an increased boost in sales, as the uncertain nature of generic versions entering the market has been stalled, leaving Nexium as one of the more popular options for consumers.

The power of profit dominates the pharmaceutical industry. This can be seen through the limited availability of affordable prescription drugs in the

United States. The average retail prices of brand-name drugs for consumers are more than triple the cost of generic versions, as prices for prescriptions increased more than three times the inflation rate from 1998 to 2000 ("Prescription drug trends" 2007). The FDA is what is called a "captured agency," being accused of serving the brand-name drug manufacturers first and foremost, as the FDA's existence relies on the presence of the pharmaceutical industry itself. Without the pharmaceutical drug industry, simply stated, the FDA would not need to exist. The FDA's existence relies not only on the presence, but the success, of the pharmaceutical drug sector. Horwitz has written on the influence of such an industry in association with its regulatory agency. Where other theories show that regulatory agencies can have merely an influence over industries, "capture theory" shows how the relationship between the FDA and the brand-name drug sector is based on mutual dependence. As Horwitz's capture theory asserts, agencies are taken over, or captured, by regulated industries. Capture is an influence model as well, but the strength and completeness of this influence makes it qualitatively different. The implication [of capture theory] is that a captured agency [the FDA, author's emphasis] systematically favors the private interests of regulated parties [pharmaceutical companies, author's emphasis] and systematically ignores the public interest (Horwitz 1989). In this sense, rather than protecting the interests of the public, meaning that the health and safety of individual patients is made a priority, the FDA has been systematically designed to simultaneously protect and benefit the pharmaceutical drug sector.

By extending manufacturer exclusivity to the brand-name sector, these drugs are marketed toward consumers as (apparently) the only option when visiting their physician. Patients then identify with these brand names and tend to request them by name once brand recognition has taken place. Although generic medications are widely used in the United States, comprising 63% of all prescriptions written, there is still much work to be done in terms of alleviating high health care costs ("Prescription drug trends" 2007). Research suggests that by replacing brand-name medications in the United States with biomolecular equivalents (generic forms), overall drug spending in the United States could be reduced by 11% (Haas et al. 2005).

THE CONTENT OF DTC ADVERTISEMENTS

This political economy analysis has shown that the interconnected relationships in the pharmaceutical industry in the United States may be influencing the ways in which advertisements are regulated and healthcare information is disseminated. The logics of capital dominate the healthcare industry, perhaps resulting in consumers being uninformed and misinformed regarding less-effectively monetized generics. If consumers are not informed regarding other options, they may simultaneously become less aware of their specific needs. The focus becomes more on finding a product that is simply reliable and serves a general purpose, as opposed to finding a product that is suited more for individual qualities (Scitovsky 1971). One goal of the pharmaceutical industry, in fact, is to keep the consumer uninformed to their full range of drug and treatment options. In an uninformed market, a consumer is not equipped to make the most rational choices. As a result of this, the consumers become unable to demand the right kind of information (Scitovsky 1971). Scitovsky explained that this is why advertising in the uninformed market relies on emotional appeal, because it leaves the buyer as uninformed as they were prior to viewing the advertisement. Emotional appeals distract consumers from the most important factual features of the product, thus keeping them less educated regarding potential medication risks (Scitovsky 1971). The pharmaceutical industry has been successful in utilizing emotional appeals in its marketing efforts rather than emphasizing these advertisements as sources of medical information for consumers, but DTCA is not without its advocates.

Two primary schools of thought exist in relation to DTCA. Proponents for the advertisements argue they have the ability to educate the public about health conditions and available treatments, essentially offering empowerment for individuals to become more involved in their health care (Holmer 1999). Understandably, medicine and pharmaceutical options are areas that have the ability to confuse individuals, and pharmaceutical advertisements theoretically have the ability to educate individuals on possible health conditions and subsequent treatment options. This is to say that prescription drugs are extremely valuable for society – they allow individuals to function better every day, and they have become a necessary aspect of Western medicine. If executed correctly, pharmaceutical advertisements may actually help to keep health care costs down by creating a more competitive marketplace. However, in an area that often can be overwhelming to individuals, these promotions may seem as offering "power to the powerless," prompting a belief that desires in their life may be fulfilled if a particular drug is consumed (e.g. more wealth, better relationships, more friends, etc.), yet, this is not necessary for one to be more proactive in discussing health care options with a health care provider. A question this book seeks to address is whether this is a false sense of power, ultimately creating a sense of pseudo-autonomy to turn consumers into patients via the process of pharmaceutical fetishism.

Critics of DTCA claim that these advertisements mislead consumers, prompting them to want products they may not need or that may be more expensive than other remedies, such as simple lifestyle changes

(Hollon 1999). Historically, the point of advertisements has been to sell products, increasing a bottom line for profit-making potential, so the argument that an advertisement is meant to educate a consumer seems to conflict with capitalist interests.

One mitigating factor is consumers' perceptions that advertising's persuasion may affect others, but not them. One study using in-depth interviews with older adults (ages 65 and older) focused on individual perceptions of DTC advertisements. The results suggested that a third person effect was found in the majority of interviews with older adults, meaning that respondents perceived DTC advertisements as having the potential to influence others more than themselves (DeLorme, Huh, and Reid 2007). Interviewees felt that others were more likely than themselves to become aware of new health conditions or medication options, ask their physician about a specific drug, and abuse prescription drugs (DeLorme, Huh, and Reid 2007). This study suggests that, in terms of persuasiveness, individuals may believe they are not susceptible to advertising tactics present in the prescription drug market, especially when accompanied by personality (viewing another person as gullible or a hypochondriac), and/or message factors (presented with an unbalanced presentation of drug benefits and risks) (DeLorme, Huh, and Reid 2007).

What might previous research tell us about the nature of DTCA? Much valuable work has been done on DTCA, but it is not a complete portrait. For example, there is a presence of a "medium bias" in the literature. The majority of research conducted in relation to DTC advertisements has focused on content analyses of print advertisements (Abel, Lee, and Weeks 2007; Bell, Kravitz, and Wilkes 1999; Holmes and Desselle 2004; Mastin et al. 2007; Welch Cline and Young 2004). Broadcast advertisements, however, have further reach than print versions, often being featured during primetime programming on television. Broadcast advertisements are arguably more symbolically complex given the modalities of video, graphics and sound, creating nuances in actors, settings, animation, background music, and narration.

A few studies focusing on broadcast formats do exist, and in such cases an emphasis is on emotional versus rational appeals in DTC advertisements; in fact, this characterizes much of the work on print advertising as well. Main, Argo, and Huhman (2004) found that emotional appeals were used far more than informative appeals, with one third of the advertisements relying on informative techniques, and two thirds of the advertisements using persuasive techniques. Another, arguably more influential, broadcast DTC advertisement study was conducted by Frosch et al. (2007), using a larger sample and number of variables in order to determine whether pharmaceutical advertisements from a 2004 sample made accurate and useful factual claims about the conditions they were treating. This study is important because a point of contention with DTCA, as discussed earlier, is whether advertisements serve as a form of education or persuasion for consumers. Frosch et al. (2007) found that the majority of prescription drug advertisements from their sample (82%) made factual claims about the condition a drug was designed to treat, yet few described condition causes (26%), risk factors for a condition (26%), or prevalence (25%). The study also found that emotional appeals (i.e. fear or happiness) were nearly universal (95%), with the ability to regain control as a result of taking the medication (85%) as a major theme.

How people appear in DTC advertisements may be designed to trigger emotional responses. Welch Cline and Young (2004) conducted a content analysis of all DTCA found in 18 popular magazines from January 1998 to December 1999 (featuring 994 DTC advertisements for 83 unique drugs), coding for: the use of models, identity rewards, and relational rewards. Identity rewards included whether models appeared to be healthy, active, or friendly, and relational rewards included social context (family, romantic, work, recreational, or other) and relational context (individual alone, dyad interaction, or group of more than two people).

Although the informational content of DTC advertisements is extremely important for making educated health care decisions, it may not be the most important feature when compared with identity and relational rewards associated with products, as these components can act as forms of observational learning for individuals (Welch Cline and Young 2004). The results showed that 91.8% of advertisements depicted exclusively healthy appearing individuals, 60.4% depicted identity-rewarding levels of activity (with physical activity occurring most frequently), and 72% of ads depicted at least one person smiling (Welch Cline and Young 2004). Overall, 96.7% of the advertisements depicted at least one identity reward, showing the ways in which even a print version of an advertisement can present strong visual cues for consumers.

Schooler, Basil, and Altman (1996) found that, in billboard advertisements, consumers were exposed to identity and relational motivators, both of which contribute to forms of social learning. Specifically, billboards for alcohol and cigarettes featured more forms of social modeling than any other products, with identity motivators being defined as using more attractiveness cues and relational motivators featuring social rewards as a result of product use. This means that having the ability to symbolically associate value with a medication goes beyond basic conceptions of health, whereas controlling a condition becomes synonymous with controlling one's identity (Charmaz 1991).

The aforementioned research suggests that DTCA attracts the attention of consumers not by offering informational content of a prescription drug, but instead by focusing on messages that invite a particular identification with depictions, associate rewards with these depictions, and thereby suggest that a reward can be gained by obtaining a particular advertised drug (Welch Cline and Young 2004). Being that research has shown the potential for observational learning that DTC advertisements feature, it is all the more important to look critically at the content of these advertisements in an effort to further understand exactly what types of messages are being promoted to consumers.

Infusing emotional situations with rhetorical appeals designed to heighten the emotional impact of an advertisement (and its subsequent interpretation by the consumer) is certainly problematic if not outright deceptive, suggesting a dubious relationship between advertising's ostensible and actual intent. There is also the potential for patients to see these advertisements as a "quick-fix" for health ailments, leading them to believe that one pill can provide a remedy without encouraging serious consideration of potential side effects or risks. This point is clarified through a content analysis conducted in 2004, which found that consumers were given more time to digest information about the benefits of a drug than associated risks (Kaphingst et al. 2004). This same study found that the benefits of a drug were delivered to suit a lower grade level of literacy (sixth grade), whereas the side effects presented are more suited for a higher grade level of literacy (ninth grade) in order to be comprehended by consumers (Kaphingst et al. 2004). Such findings suggest that, rather than educating consumers on drugs and their potential side effects and risks, advertisers prioritize revenue over social responsibility, an especially serious concern given that prescription drugs can cause serious health hazards, and in the most serious of cases, death.

THE EFFECTS OF DTCA

Other research has focused on the potential persuasive effectiveness of DTC advertisements. One of the largest studies conducted regarding consumer comprehension found that, of 2,653 respondents taken from a demographically balanced national sample, 32% reported having read or listened to most prescription drug advertisements (Beltramini 2006). Over 50% reported wanting to ask their doctor for more information about a prescription upon viewing or hearing an advertisement, with 53% eventually reporting visiting their doctor (with 39% of these individuals receiving the prescription upon asking their doctor for it) (Beltramini 2006).

Kravitz et al. (2005) conducted a randomized controlled trial to examine prescribing rates of physicians in response to drug requests by patients after they had viewed DTC advertisements. Unannounced visits to 152 primary care physicians were made by women actors that were randomized to one of three behaviors: requests for an advertised antidepressant (Paxil), a general unbranded request, or no request at all. The study found that more than 50%

of physicians felt the patients had correctly diagnosed themselves based on the DTC advertisement alone, with the patients that requested Paxil by name receiving the antidepressant 53% of the time for depression and 55% of the time for adjustment disorder (Kravitz et al. 2005). These findings point to the effectiveness of DTC advertisements, meaning that examining their content and its implications are important considerations as well.

Not only is DTCA ubiquitous, but studies have suggested that a majority of people believe the ads themselves are truthful and give them hope for their treatment options. Nearly 70% of people questioned in 2001 believed that DTC advertisements provided enough information to make a good health care decision, yet 60% did not feel that the advertisements gave enough information about the risks or side effects (Gellad and Lyles 2007). Scholars have suggested that this fact becomes problematic because the way DTC advertisements are regulated leaves the pharmaceutical company, which is a corporation with a responsibility to its bottom line, holding a large amount of the power to determine how to frame the particular health care message. Looking more closely at the ways in which the presentation of benefits versus risks in an advertisement could impact an individual is important. If consumers are not given fair and balanced information, how can they be expected to make the most informed decision with the physician?

A 2001 study by the Kaiser Family Foundation looked at the effect of DTC advertisements on consumers. The study found that, overall, 13% of adults in the United States have at some point in their lifetime received a prescription drug from a physician after seeing a prescription drug advertisement (Anderson 2003). Of the adult population sampled, 30% had talked to their physicians about specific DTC advertisements they had seen, and of that 30%, 44% had received a prescription for the drug they had inquired about (Anderson 2003). Public awareness of DTCA has increased significantly since the FDA's Modernization Act in 1997. Prior to the amendment taking effect, in 1997, 63% of adults recalled seeing pharmaceutical advertisements. By 2002, 85% had reported being aware of these advertisements (Anderson 2003). Research has shown that by the year 2011, over 50% of patient requests made to physicians for a drug as a result of viewing a DTC advertisement were granted, meaning that these advertisements are influential, to say the least (Ventola 2011).

Studies have also looked at physician attitudes toward DTCA. According to a 2013 study conducted by the FDA, 63% of physicians themselves have reported that DTCA misinforms patients, with 74% believing that DTC advertisements overemphasize the benefits of a drug (Meyer 2013). Especially problematic is the perceived safety of advertised prescription drugs, with 68% of doctors agreeing that prescription drugs are marketed well-before safety profiles can be obtained (Meyer 2013). As physicians have reported that DTCA has negative effects in terms of self-diagnosis, research has supported this claim by looking at the effects of observational learning in health care advertisements, specifically those promoting prescription drugs.

Despite much solid content work on DTCA, arguably there are areas to still be explored. Two such limitations were previously discussed: emphases on print DTC advertisements and a fairly circumscribed range of persuasive appeals in the ads. Another is the use of one method – in most cases, the method being quantitative in nature. Mixed-methods analyses are not common within this literature, most often utilizing either quantitative or qualitative approaches (Faerber and Kreling 2014; Frosch et al. 2007; Gooblar and Carpenter 2013; Kaphingst et al. 2004; Yang et al. 2012). Quantitative research has a much larger presence (Faerber and Kreling 2014; Frosch et al. 2007; Kaphingst et al. 2004; Yang et al. 2012) and when qualitative frameworks are used, analyses are most often performed on a historical level, tracing the FDA's role in pharmaceutical advertising and presenting both sides of the "pharmaceutical advertising debate." Although highly important, few critical works on DTCA as presenting limited courses of health prevention have been published (Landau 2011; Quesinberry Stokes 2013).

Given the above limitations of the literature – a narrow range of research questions dealing with factual claims and accuracy, a focus on print advertisements, and uni-dimensional approaches to methods – it becomes necessary to update and replicate earlier quantitative measures of DTC advertisements (most notably Frosch et al. 2007), while expanding the conversation that considers how these advertisements impact society. In the case of DTCA, a mixed-methods approach is useful because quantitative content analysis can present a strong foundation (via findings) to paint a basic statistical picture regarding the current state of prescription drug advertisements, which can then be more deeply and qualitatively analyzed in order to discuss the implications associated with more critical concepts such as medicalization and pharmaceuticalization, as shown through prominent examples and rich qualitative description. Qualitative analysis can shed light on the implications for meaning-making these advertisements have for consumers. By more descriptively presenting and discussing the content of these advertisements, what types of individuals are being represented can better be explored. For example, are there significant patterns in terms of gender, race, socioeconomic status, etc. being shown? Furthermore, how are patients being portrayed? If individuals are shown as being active, healthy, and happy during the majority of these advertisements, then these traits are being sold alongside a product, influencing an individual's choice to speak with their doctor about beginning a medication regimen.

Critical-cultural orientations to media typically engage such issues as social power, meaning construction, ideology and hegemony. Conversations surrounding DTCA research must be expanded to include how pharmaceutical companies are shaping the meaning of drug interventions for individuals in the United States from a critical perspective, including the ways in which DTC advertisements frame issues of identity and representation for patients and health care in advertising. Such issues highlight the ways in which patients are being framed as consumers in advertisements, which then permits the commodification of health care to be celebrated. Such a celebration has ideological implications, including definitions of "the good life," patient agency and the role of DTC advertisements in such depictions. Literature on DTCA has presented it as a category separate from other advertising and forms of consumer culture, seeing that these forms of advertising focus on a product that is particularly unique – patients can only obtain the product through a third party, or gatekeeper, which is the physician. It certainly is true that such ads have unique qualities, including a heavily regulatory environment and a targeted consumer who cannot directly purchase a product without a physician's consent. Critical theory that studies DTC advertisements should understand the unique nature of medical commodities. To accomplish this, the perspective of "medicalization" – a perspective that critically analyzes the increased application of a traditional medical model to a variety of problems – will be applied to DTCA.

In addition, however, DTC advertisements are by definition forms of branded product advertising. Thus, common ideological tendencies are shared between DTC advertisements and the textual genre of advertisements overall; this perspective toward DTC advertisements has been underdeveloped. By positioning this work from a critical advertising studies perspective that highlights such elements as class, race, gender, and commodification, an important commercial context can be emphasized and deconstructed. To the point, while DTC advertisements are unique in nature because of what is being sold to consumers, this does not mean that the content present is insusceptible to traditional patterns seen throughout advertising as a whole. For this reason, this book seeks to develop a critical analysis of how patients and aspects of life are framed in these advertisements, which can then help to explain increased instances of medicalization, and perhaps more precisely, "pharmaceuticalization," in the United States.

Chapter 2

Theoretical Foundations

Important Approaches to DTCA

The previous chapter concluded by arguing for a critical approach toward health communication research as a crucial component for understanding how heath care treatment options, consumers, and elements of life generally are framed by the media and advertising industries. This book relies on several theoretical foundations, but the main theoretical underpinnings come from more critical trajectories as seen in Critical Advertising Studies, as this project is seeking to explicate the ways in which pharmaceutical advertisements act as a form of commodified portrayals of health care and what it means for people to be proactive in their own health care treatment. Whereas the previous section addressed one important component of the Critical Advertising Studies perspective toward research (the production processes and economics involved within the industry), this chapter seeks to address another important facet of the issue: texts (pharmaceutical advertisements) as having meaning-making abilities for individuals. Such meaning-making is not neutral, however, and is embedded in issues of power inequities.

CRITICAL ADVERTISING STUDIES

Advertising can be defined as any form of promotional culture involving three important aspects: payment for time or space by advertisers, a clear demarcation of its presence as an advertisement and the involvement of an advertiser, and a persuasive component that urges an individual to take a form of action by means of "argument, reasoning, or emotional plea" (Turow and McAllister 2009, 2). Advertising is prominent in helping to create consumer culture, which involves the symbols and messages surrounding individuals and the process of meaning-making invoked by these messages (Turow and McAllister 2009).

Critical Advertising Studies is part of the larger paradigm of critical-cultural media studies. Critical approaches to culture were seen as early as the 1920s through work from the Frankfurt School, which by the 1930s included theorists Horkheimer, Adorno, Fromm, Marcuse, Lowenthal, and Benjamin (Kellner and Durham 2012). Such work began the critical tradition of exploring how media perpetuates or challenges social and cultural inequities. The Frankfurt School, strongly influenced by the works of Karl Marx and contextualized by the rise of both fascism and industrial capitalism, examined popular culture through the lens of media as a powerful creator, emphasizing the media's subsequent repression of other economic and cultural forces that could lead to social change and true progressive thought. One of the most influential essays by Horkheimer and Adorno, originally written in the 1940s (reprinted in 2002), focused on both the standardizing and narcotizing elements of mass culture, but also the entrenchment of advertising as a cultural form. Horkheimer and Adorno's *The Culture Industry: Enlightenment as Mass Deception* analyzes the mass industrialization imposed on cultural production as a totalizing system where culture is structured to benefit the larger cultural industry, and functions by disallowing the potential for human individuality, yet this piece repeatedly emphasizes that the existence of human individuality in modern industrialized culture is a myth (Horkheimer and Adorno 1972). Rather, the culture industry promotes forms of pseudo-individuality in which trivial differences are falsely offered as genuine options for life decisions, therefore co-opting true individuality.

Admittedly, the deterministic ontology of Horkheimer and Adorno's work leads to the assumption that individuals do not have agency or an ability to create "true meaning" from their media and the work has been much criticized for a totalizing view of an oppressive cultural system. An interesting point is the title of this work, emphasizing the singular cultural "industry" as opposed to "industries," noting that economic coercion has only given society one option. While our ideology says that we have the freedom to choose, in reality, we have only the freedom to choose from what is the same, coming from one industry alone (Horkheimer and Adorno 1972). This essay has two especially notable points. First, the Frankfurt School scholars emphasize processes of standardization in their writing, as they are seeing similar trends in Western media which they had seen in the fascist media from which they came in Germany. The standardization of culture creates a uniformity of style and ideas, meaning that when one is constantly exposed to sameness, the ability to question and offer true critique becomes blunted. Second, this essay is a very early example of advertising criticism, as the industrialized nature of media at the time had made it an ideal conduit for advertising.

The routine schedule of advertising (30-minute long programs with periodic commercial breaks, with new programs beginning on the hour) allows a scheduling template for "art" to be presented to individuals, whereby they are consistently getting the message that a product will improve life (a point to be later emphasized by other scholars, including Raymond Williams); however, once one acquires a product, little ever changes (Horkheimer and Adorno 1972). Horkheimer and Adorno stress the importance of advertising in creating pseudo-individuality for society at the end of their essay, stating that the triumph of advertising is its ability to urge consumers to compulsively imitate the images they see in advertising, where a freedom to choose from products becomes a freedom to be the same as everyone else given the uniformity in consumer culture (Horkheimer and Adorno 1972).

Later movements in cultural studies such as the University of Birmingham Centre for Contemporary Cultural Studies, created in 1964, and directed by Stuart Hall in 1968, added the importance of studying specific symbolic and semiotic elements of popular culture to track how ideologies were constructed and challenged in popular culture. The Birmingham group provided a wide variety of critical-cultural perspectives and was among the first to study how audiences may be influenced by the cultural meanings in mass communications, especially the representation of ideology, class, gender, and race in cultural texts (Kellner and Durham 2012). An influential theorist for the Birmingham Centre was Raymond Williams, who wrote a much-cited essay on the history and symbolic logic of advertising.

In order to describe the subfield that is called Critical Advertising Studies, it is helpful to briefly trace the history of pivotal changes in production and consumption from a Western perspective. While the subfield's history is rich, a brief analysis of its roots allows for a deeper understanding of scholarly concerns and questions. A general increase in advertising came as a result of the Industrial Revolution, with both increases in production and business-friendly policies playing key roles: in England the abolition of the Advertising Tax in 1853 allowed creative industries to change the landscape of consumer culture (Williams 1980). Advances in mass production from 1880–1920 emphasized a more standardized system of distribution, alongside an evolution in the household – with the advent of new products and technologies, domestic routines became more about purchasing and less about "doing," creating new ways for individuals to relate to the objects sold on the idea of making their lives easier (Strasser 2009). Advertising filled a void for educating consumers on new products they knew nothing about. Beyond providing information on these new products, advertisements were able to "teach" buyers a set of values and norms in the developing age of consumer culture, giving generations the "tools" (branded commodities) to create their identities (Strasser 1989). Image-oriented magazine advertising constructed branded images on a national scale by the end of the 1800s. Radio advertising, beginning in the late 1920s, added such persuasive techniques as jingles and vocal qualities to the branding arsenal.

There was resistance however. Stuart Chase and F. J. Schlink's Your Money's Worth: A Study in the Waste of the Consumer's Dollars (1927) was one of the first catalysts for consumer activists objecting to advertising practices, as the authors exposed propaganda techniques used by the industry. Public outcry prompted the Roosevelt administration to call for federal regulation of advertising, leading to the Food and Drug Act which gave the Food and Drug Administration the authority to ban an advertisement for any food, drug, or cosmetic if it provided false information (Stole 2013). However, as World War II spread throughout Europe in the 1940s, the U.S. government approached the advertising community, requesting help with promotional materials to educate the public on its war efforts (also referred to as propaganda campaigns). It was at this point that political debates concerning advertising began to minimize, as the industry used this opportunity to build the nation's morale while simultaneously acting as a primary public information service (Stole 2013). A new wave of consumer activism came in the 1960s and 1970s with the discovery of fraud against consumers, largely creating a critical public view of the industry (Cross 2013). Over the years, joining these voices of criticism were critical advertising scholars.

In its current manifestation, Critical Advertising Studies emphasizes two main areas of research: advertising as a cultural system and advertising as a funding system (McAllister and West 2013). Advertising as a cultural system involves looking at such issues as representation in advertising and how advertising offers a commodity as a solution to a social or personal problem (McAllister and West 2013). Issues of representation could include gender (Goffman 1979), race, class, able-bodiedness, and nationality, among others. In such cases, scholars address how advertising contributes to cultural constructions of social identity; such identities are embedded in power relations and are at their heart ideological. Advertising was seen, then, not just as a form of persuasion for short-term goals (selling a brand), but also as a symbol system that generated media beyond the selling function.

Significant scholarship has addressed advertising representation, often focusing on attempts by companies to capitalize on market segments while presenting extremely limited notions of diversity (Dines and Humez 2015). For example, critical research has analyzed the circumscribed role of women in advertisements. Women in advertising are often portrayed as overtly feminine, yet even notions of femininity become very limited. This means that women in advertising are often portrayed as being dependent on others, having a fixation on beauty, positioning them in roles that emphasize family and nurturing, and having a fear of technology (Steinem 2003). Others note the focus on traditional gender roles such as the housewife or mother (Hollows 2003). By encoding modern conceptions of female identity in advertising, it can be clearly seen how this identity is largely created based on the construction of women as consumers (Friedan 1963). Conversely, critical approaches toward advertising have looked at how male consumers are represented as overly masculine, including the Depression-era creations of masculinity in ads used to sell idealized versions of self-identification during a challenging economic time (Breazeale 1994). Representations of masculinity in advertisements feature a simultaneous exploitation and denial of the feminine, meaning that male consumers are framed via women – notions of masculinity are perpetuated by positioning men in advertisements alongside women that are represented as servicing men, not only on a sexual level, but via markers of class as well (Breazeale 1994). While representations regarding the role of women in advertisements and notions of femininity/masculinity have been addressed in critical advertising literature, research has yet to fully address the nuances of these portrayals as they are depicted via DTCA, creating a current gap in the existing literature.

With representations of older adults in advertisements, when such representations are the main focus of the ads, the actors/models used almost always look physically young and attractive in appearance (Carrigan and Szmigin 2002). By creating and perpetuating images that feature older adults as youthful, downplaying the challenges associated with growing older, advertising frames older adults as illegitimate members of society (Carrigan and Szmigin 2002). These images encourage older adults to be seen as young, strong, independent, and sexy – all while experiencing increased health problems and facing retirement, which itself is represented as signifying a loss of functioning and income for individuals. When coupled with advertising's already inherent expectations of youth, fitness, and beauty, the result is a new set of exclusions for older adults (Chaney 1995). Again, research has yet to explicate the ways in which DTC advertisements portray older adults, and whether these representations are consistent with the existing literature described above.

When looking at advertising as a funding system, a political economy approach is used to look its production and distribution of culture when the culture depends upon advertising revenue to finance its media systems, acknowledging that a specific set of relationships between economy, social institutions, organizations, and media influence cultural meanings. Western scholarship emphasizes how capitalism structures modes of production and social practices according to the logic of commodification, emphasizing a profit imperative (Kellner and Durham 2012); advertising and advertising-supported media are implicated in such structures. A political economy approach, such as that conducted in this chapter, interrogates the content and implications of commercial ideology and its relationship to existing structures of power and privilege, while also looking at how ideology is produced within the organizational and occupational framework of media industries (Jhally and Livant 1990). Commercial ideology, then, is not just a product of advertising messages, but may infuse many media messages with consumerist views. As Schiller (1992) described, Western industrialized society has replaced family, religion, and education with media as a traditional form of socialization, creating an "ideology of consumerism" that is researched in Critical Advertising Studies. One of the most important aspects to analyze alongside ideologies of consumption is the concept of commodity fetishism, as this term explicates the ways in which advertising attempts to influence the meanings of goods for individuals and, critical scholars argue, elevate the social status of these goods while simultaneously decontextualizing them.

COMMODITY FETISHISM

Commodity fetishism is a process whereby the process of commodification constructs in particular ways the understanding of processes of production, as advertising and brand discourse ignore how products are created and rather emphasize additional meaning or symbolic agency around brands for consumers (McAllister 2014). Commodity fetishism mitigates the relationship between people and manufactured commodities, and fetishism occurs once individuals see meaning in things as inherent part of their physical existence, seemingly removing the labor and social processes involved in the production of the commodity (Marx 1992).

The work of Raymond Williams (1980) segues well with commodity fetishism. Williams' seminal work, originally written in the 1960s, outlines advertising and public relations practices that are still influential today. The most prominent aspect to come out of his essay "Advertising: The Magic System" are the conceptions of advertising as "magic," referring to the ability of advertising to go beyond the material and appeal to the desires of individuals (Williams 1980). A common claim about consumer culture, Williams argues, is that modern consumers are very materialistic: we are driven by the need to acquire material goods for their own sake. But he posits that advertising works the way it does because individuals are, in fact, not materialist enough, as members of society are not satisfied with the material product, but require an additional, secondary effect (e.g. clothing must only serve its functional purpose, but it also has the ability to make us feel popular, sexy, happy, etc.) (Williams 1980). If individuals were purely materialistic, advertisements would only need to display the commodities themselves; a new commodity would be the only motivation consumers need. Instead, individuals are driven by other values besides the material: love, belongingness, security, for example. They thus look for added meaning or value in products, a dilemma given the high level of standardization in product categories. Thus, advertising works by promising to fulfill additional needs and desires that go beyond the material using highly evocative and emotional symbols. The magic, then, is that advertising tells us our desires can be met by purchasing the product. Just as the production context of modern commodities is removed by the industrialization process, Williams work reminds us that advertising adds new meanings to commodities to fill that meaning gap.

Much of Williams' argument relies on the Marxist concepts of use-value and exchange-value as they relate to commodity fetishism. The use-value of a commodity refers to its material value. For example, the use-value of clothing is to cover and protect the body. The exchange-value, however, becomes much more difficult to identify, and can often be attributed to capital, but it is more abstract than this. Exchange-value increases as the labor it takes to create a commodity increases, and exchange-value rests on the notion that two commodities can be exchanged in an open market as they are always being compared to a third facet functioning as their "universal equivalent" (most often times money) (Marx 1992). An understanding of the relationship between use-value and exchange-value of commodities allows advertising to be better understood as a form of relating people with objects. Advertisements, including those for pharmaceuticals, allow for culture to associate products with additional meaning, as emotional meaning, forms of promotional culture, and even packaging designs evoke sentiment for individuals (Williams 1980). When such meanings enhance the use of value of a commodity (a sports car equals prestige, for example), it may also enhance its exchange-value in the marketplace.

An important work to consider when describing commodity fetishism is Sut Jhally's expansion upon Dallas Smythe's work from the 1970s, which argues for a political economic lens when addressing advertising and its relationships to audiences. Jhally attempts to trace how the media's use of advertising acts as a mediator between cultural understanding and a capitalist economy (Jhally 1990). Jhally considers two concepts most important when studying the field of advertising. First, he emphasizes the fetishism of commodities, as defined by Marx, citing the advertising industry's creation of additional qualities for products beyond their material use. Here, he describes the "reading" of goods as necessary for understanding their commodity form. By doing so, we can better explain the social relations of production and how these relations are reflected in goods themselves. By focusing on the fetishism of commodities, in this case, pharmaceuticals, this book can explicate how our capitalist system empties these commodities of their "real" meaning, or use-value (serving as a remedy for a health ailment). This, then, permits pharmaceutical advertising to insert meaning into the relationship between health and prescription drugs for consumers – as the use-value becomes subsumed by exchange-value for the manufacturers of such drugs, and as use-value becomes expanded for consumers beyond their immediate medicinal qualities to those involving happiness and "the good life." Just as DTCA requests labor on behalf of individual consumers by encouraging them to personally connect with an advertisement, it is evident that consumers are simultaneously performing different types of labor that directly benefit the pharmaceutical industry as a whole.

A SMYTHIAN ANALYSIS: DTCA CONSUMERS AS LABORERS

Credited with igniting the "blind spot debate" in 1977, Dallas Smythe considers two important metaphors in his important piece *On the Audience Commodity and Its Work*: audience as commodity and audience as labor. Smythe dismisses the idea that media are best studied by analyzing texts to discover the ideology that produces society's consciousness. He claims that the "blind spot" of Western Marxism involves its dismissal of media industries and he provides his own theory that the media are central to Marxist concepts, manufacturing only one commodity: the audience (Meehan 2002). In this sense, media industries are assembling and selling audiences to advertisers, leaving content and programming as a secondary "free lunch" (Smythe 1980).

By media industries selling their audiences to advertisers, the implication is that advertisers want to maximize the utility of this commodity. Audiences give their attention and time, being paid through content other than the advertisement (thus referring to the free lunch), and Smythe says that audiences are in fact working when they watch these advertisements, with their payment being the television content itself (Smythe 1980). There is an additional work performed by the audience as they incorporate these products into their leisure time, so individuals are also laboring whenever a product or advertisement is part of their consciousness. As Smythe considers audience time as a form of labor, he claims that television is always asking viewers to be working, interpolating individuals as "consumer-oriented laborers" that integrate products seen in advertisements into their everyday lives. Smythe also critiques the media industries for cheating on their payment to audiences by requiring them to accept the cost of buying the equipment needed for content – televisions, radios, cable bills, electric bills, and so on. Advertising affects the logic of programming also, as the programs often being watched are television shows structured around advertising, including messages that promote consumption and product placement (Smythe 1980). Beyond these forms of labor, this book argues that an important form of work being performed by consumers of DTCA relates to the meaning-making abilities of advertisements. Consumers are responsible for adding, or at least solidifying, meaning to prescription drugs being advertised once they inquire about these brands with their physicians. By utilizing signifiers and signifying practices that reveal underlying dimensions of a possible autonomy for a patient, DTCA acts as a mechanism that essentially leaves consumers blind, as their request for specific brands of prescription drugs when meeting with physicians essentially leaves them blinded to their aiding in masking the role of drug companies if they act in the ways these advertisements suggest they should.

According to Smythe (1980), advertising has the power to do multiple things. First, it places value on audiences, labeling them as "demographics," and giving some audiences more value than others. It also impacts the quantity of content, often accelerating the pace of media. Advertisements have to be flashy and entertaining in order to receive audience attention, so television content must do the same in order to keep up with the industry. Advertising also trivializes content, allowing audiences to take their media less seriously. Above all else, advertising provides society with less critical media coverage, as media industries take a pro-advertising stance and often integrate products in their coverage. The idea of audience as commodity is built into our logic of traditional and new media, with new media being dependent on audiences for its existence. Audiences can now be media creators themselves, which simultaneously provides data points about their identities to advertising researchers (Smythe 1980).

A "Smythian" analysis in the context of DTCA is appropriate, as consumers are doing "work" by engaging with the advertisements, thinking about the meanings of brands and talking about them with their friends and family. In addition, beyond participating in the work involved to pay attention to these forms of promotion, with DTC advertisements, consumers take the additional steps of visiting a physician to ask about a particular drug or request it outright. In this sense, DTCA is an industry that requires its viewing audience to become labor-performing consumers themselves, seeing that by asking a physician about a drug, they essentially become a new form of promotion for the drug itself, further "advocating" to a physician their willingness to consume. The logic of the system of DTCA, then, is that consumers are molded into salespersons for these drugs, ultimately becoming the main sales force, as these advertisements become an intermediary between physicians and patients.

Critical Advertising Studies and commodity fetishism aide in the development of DTCA research particularly in its ability to address the pharmaceutical industry's impact on the meaning-making practices of individuals – but also addresses implications beyond purely persuasive appeals – and how consumers are encouraged to conceptualize health in a very particular way, most often while being offered a sense of pseudo-individuality and pseudo-autonomy. The theoretical foundations and social processes from Critical Advertising Studies and commodity fetishism can be combined with those of two other theoretical concepts – medicalization and pharmaceuticalization – to critique the nuances present in the content of DTC advertisements.

MEDICALIZATION: A HISTORICAL EXPLANATION AND A CONSUMERIST DISCOURSE PERSPECTIVE

Although numerous key stakeholders comprise the field of health care, patients and citizens invested in their health, in particular, have been the group that have been most affected by changes in the organization of health care, transitions in the acquisition of medical knowledge, and volatile market events. Much of the dilemma in understanding such changes and the citizen's role in them involves how changes and current health structures and practices are articulated. An analysis of professional health care thus requires an approach emphasizing discursive practices in order to learn how the cultural practices and meanings of health are produced and understood. Discourse can be understood broadly as a series of symbolized actions, not merely representations, which further constitute and solidify cultural logics and practices; critical-cultural work emphasizes the understanding of such discursive constructions, including ones that are multi-modal, narrativized, and offer constructions of multiple health care elements, as is the case with U.S. pharmaceutical advertisements. But such health discourses are embedded in a history of social constructions and institutional dynamic involving western medicine. One notably important historical dynamic is medicalization, a concept associated with work from several disciplines.

Especially influential in the medicalization literature is Michel Foucault. First published in 1963, Foucault's The Birth of the Clinic traces changes in medicine, the medical profession, and the clinic (referencing teaching hospitals), focusing primarily on the social and political changes brought about after the French Revolution in 1789. The central theme of Foucault's work is his conception of the "clinical gaze" (or medical gaze), which can be partly summarized as the separation by the medical profession of the patient, whereby the body becomes a separate unit from an individual's identity or being (Foucault 1994). Foucault reflects on important historical events or shifts in order to analyze the structures of medicine, treating each as a discursive system, insisting that medical discourse is action and not merely representation (Foucault 1983). Foucault's key objective is to address the processes by which cultural and scientific meanings of the medical profession have been produced and understood over time (Long 1992).

Foucault is adamant in his description of the doctor as having a political role, claiming that doctors became "politicized administrators" during the nineteenth century, making value judgments on behalf of patients about their care (Foucault 1994). Foucault's text continues by marking the point at which the discursive formulation of medical knowledge took place, citing teaching hospitals (clinics) as areas that first allowed the patient to become de-centered (Foucault 1994). At the beginning of the Renaissance period, education was seen as a positive value for enlightenment, furthering the practice of training in the medical profession as a means for acquiring knowledge (Peerson 1995). The formation of this clinical method is directly related to the medical gaze, as historically patients became viewed more as teaching objects and less as individuals. At this point, the medical gaze began to define all possible health knowledge, whereby "the intervention of techniques presenting problems of measurement, substance, or composition at the level of invisible (my emphasis) structures is rejected" (Foucault 1994). The development of the teaching clinic was pivotal in constructing the medical gaze – since the eighteenth century, clinical evidence has been obtained by a doctor gazing at a patient, rather than viewing their body as one which is holistic with personhood both in processes and experiences (Long 1992). In the clinical setting, patients become live examples of disease, classified as transitory objects that doctors merely happen to come in contact with (Machado 2012).

These insights, I argue, can be directly traced to developments in the pharmaceutical industry today, as patients are still positioned as live examples of disease, with advertisements being created and disseminated that frame consumers with idealized versions of disease or illness. The discursive construction of health can be thought of as the "systematic intersection" of two series of information (one coming from the patient, the other coming from the doctor), where the intersection reveals an individual fact, or figure of knowledge, expanding the doctor-patient relationship in a way that does not often permit knowledge of the authority to be questioned (Foucault 1994). This relates to Foucault's conception of the "epistemic change" or "epistemic break" in medical knowledge itself, where the use of corpses in teaching hospitals changed the structure of the profession and its focus. The epistemic belief in using corpses as cadavers in teaching hospitals was that it could teach a more localized form of medicine. With the introduction of these corpses, the "epistemic change" resulted in that, rather than clinicians focusing on the history of a patient and their essential being, they focused on the geography of medicine (i.e. specifically where someone's body is being affected) (Foucault 1994). This created a more nominalist approach to medicine, robbing patients of an experience with their physician that emphasized history and holistic approaches to care. Medical knowledge transformed in a way that emphasized visible problems in the bodies of patients rather than inclusive, broader approaches to care. The analysis of these localized problems by physicians meant that a new epistemology had been accepted – one that permitted the view of medicine as a discipline dependent upon the rationalized comparison of "healthy" indicators to "unhealthy" indicators to be accepted as the standard for medical knowledge (Machado 2012).

An important component of the medical gaze is its subjective and ideologically driven nature (Peerson 1995). Foucault attempts to dispel the myth that the medical gaze is subconscious on behalf of the doctor – instead, he claims that medical discourse has been reciprocated for so long that it is now commonplace for doctors to view patients as two separate beings: a set of symptoms (or a case) and an individual. As I argue, the pharmaceutical industry presents itself as a form of cultural authority equal to the physician however, viewing patients as sets of symptoms only, ultimately degrading conceptions of true individuality. This form of presentation is not unlike much of the authority and weight given to quantitative over qualitative research in the field of health communication, as more generalizable concepts are typically revered as having more insight, while the nuanced and detailed interpretations offered by highlighting the individual experiences or stories of patients in the health care settings becomes overshadowed.

While the process of medicalization is often attributed to Foucault, the theoretical roots of the concept have been strongly influenced by the sociologist Ivan Illich, who coined the theory of Social Iatrogenesis. Social Iatrogensis theorizes that the structures of medicine have created health impairments (i.e. unhappiness, social anxiety) that are made more visible to the public via socioeconomic transformations in health care (Illich 1973). This means that the proliferation of disease is exacerbated by the extension of medical categories on everyday life, and this project is seeking to explicate how pharmaceutical advertisements feature content that may contribute to this process. For example, many pharmaceutical advertisements feature individuals who have intolerance for sadness, which has increased in society alongside increased diagnoses of depression (Horwitz and Wakefield 2009).

As described, traditional views on medicalization come from the field of sociology and approach the construction of disease, highlighting how medical expansion has permitted an increased sense of control over the lives of individuals and an expanded definition of what is "illness" (Williams, Gabe, and Davis 2008). While the utilization of the theory of medicalization is important in order to describe sociological constructions of health, it is my intent to offer a mass communications/media studies approach that can focus more on the constructions of health, patients, and pharmaceutical drugs via media platforms. More traditional health communication studies have positioned medicine as a form of cultural authority that is apolitical, meaning its only existence is to improve the health of citizens (McAllister 1992).

Medicalization is an attempt to deconstruct these notions, as it highlights how medical ideology has intersected into our everyday lives, often allowing the "difficulties people have" to be transformed into illness, disease, or instances that require professional medical intervention (McAllister 1992; Engelhardt 1986). Media discourses about health and medicine can serve, then, as a source for or against medicalized definitions.

Foucault's work influenced later work on medicalization through his emphasis on the development of medicalized perspectives and discourses and the resulting solidification of power of the medical profession. Peter Conrad (2007) also addresses the discursive formation of medicalization and its implications, defining medicalization as a process where non-medical problems become defined and treated as medical problems, with the key being "definition." Medical terms must define a problem, allowing medical language to create a medical framework in order to treat a social problem with a form of medical intervention (Conrad 2007). Conrad's main point is that medicalization is a process, one that becomes enacted when phenomena become defined by medical professionals as a medical problem (Conrad 2007). Conrad traces the sociological study of medicalization to the 1970s with its relation to the medical imperialism thesis of the 1960s, as medical professionals were characterized as agents of power – symbolized by the influence of such professional-level groups as the American Medical Association – seeking to maintain their social order while limiting patients based on gender, race, and socioeconomic status. The study of medicalization shifted drastically starting in the 1990s, as the structure of health care in the United States began to privilege not only physicians, but major health care industries as well. In this sense, Conrad argues, the pharmaceutical industry has become a major stakeholder in the medicalization process, as managed care often covers prescription drugs as remedies for ailments as opposed to providing long-term psychotherapeutic interventions.

Conrad's work pays homage to Foucault's medical gaze, arguing that the process of medicalization includes the application of medical treatments and solutions to human problems, but as also including something much deeper – the social control aspects of medicalization which include discourse and subjectivity (Conrad 2007). Interestingly, Conrad also uses Foucault's medical gaze to point to one of the largest problems he currently sees in health care – the ways in which medicalization too narrowly emphasizes individual problems, while ignoring larger social and environmental effects. This seemingly has strong implications for the study at hand, suggesting, for example, that the health care system in the United States calls for individualized medical interventions in the form of prescription drugs, rather than more collective or social solutions to problems, increasing the amount of medical social control over human behavior.

The commodification of medicine, as Conrad describes, leads to a discursive process whereby patients have become synonymous with consumers. As the organization of medical care has shifted, patients have had to "shop around" for their doctors in an attempt to discover what their health insurance will cover, prompting them to act more as buyers seeking out medical services rather than patients seeking quality care. In this sense, modern capitalism and sales discourse promoting the solutions of copyright protected medical technologies and drugs have expanded medicalization. While Conrad offers great explanations of the ways in which pharmaceutical drugs enter the doctor-patient relationship, his emphasis is on the creation, promotion, and application of particular medical categories to human problems and life events (Conrad 2007).

Current representations of medical knowledge are extremely influential in shaping current understandings of activities associated with health care professions today. According to Foucault (1994), the development of the clinical field of medicine permitted a discourse to be created and perpetuated whereby the patient became an "endlessly reproducible fact" to be found in all patients suffering in a similar way. Here, the plurality of observations becomes a progressive convergence where patients become classified according to their symptoms, regardless of potential variance of symptoms in the case of each unique patient (Foucault 1994). This concept relates directly to the pharmaceutical industry's advertisements, as each advertisement is required by the FDA to list both the symptoms for which a drug can be used, and also potential side effects which may result from taking a particular drug. Beyond merely a glance, the medical gaze includes both a hearing gaze and a speaking gaze, where doctors represent a moment of balance between speech and spectacle. As patients are framed as objects, doctors are framed as authority figures with unlimited medical knowledge – as a result, the medical gaze is more than just observation, as it belongs to an individual who is supported and justified by the institution in which it works, complete with the power to make decisions and intervene in health care treatments. Foucault's work is a helpful foundation for analyzing the discursive approaches to how patients and medical professionals are framed in pharmaceutical advertisements. The medical gaze allows the pharmaceutical industry to position itself as an authority figure in medical knowledge, meaning that the industry itself has the power to see an underlying reality or "hidden truth." The "hidden truth" here is that pharmaceutical advertisements sell remedies for patients in a way that offers each consumer a sense of pseudo-individuality – in the advertisements themselves, "patients" (actors) are framed as being whole, complete individuals, more than their disease, symptoms, or medical ailment. In reality, the product being sold is meant to treat a symptom or set of symptoms, thereby dismissing the patient as an individual and ignoring their "whole self."

Beyond referencing medicine's progression away from patient-centeredness, medicalization positions the patient as an object of discourse which transforms into a subject, a formal reorganization that permits the body to become a rhetorical signifier of disease, losing at least some component of individuality (Foucault 1994). This can be interpreted as viewing the patient as a display for disease, where symptoms become more important than the ailing individual. Medicalization is more than just a process, as it also aides in defining medical knowledge within the larger field of health care. The pharmaceutical industry is successful because it does not privilege individual patients' experiences and health cases, but rather, it assumes that countless individuals can be "boxed in" to a specific type of consumer, ultimately stripping patients of their treatment options, identity, and the personal intricacies and variations of the body.

To summarize, the medical gaze can be defined as the medical perception and experience acquired by physicians following the French Revolution, yet, the medical gaze exists arguably more today than ever before (Peerson 1995). By relying on the clinic and the use of corpses combined with observation-style methods of teaching, physicians were able to observe bodies in entirely new ways, allowing theories to be dispelled and new knowledge to be discovered. This led to those in the medical profession gaining a great deal of power and privilege, leaving little room for others to challenge their findings. Throughout this process, the perspective and experience of the patient become lost in translation, as the doctor's judgment was more revered. The patient, then, enters a never-ending pattern of objectification, and this objectification is exacerbated by the dividing nature of social compartmentalization (Long 1992). This objectification can be seen in the DTCA industry's positioning of the patient in forms of marketing, as patients are featured as having control and authority over the health care decisions – yet, upon deeper analysis, these forms of autonomy are false, as prescription drugs cannot offer the necessarily and exclusive remedies for all of the categories for which they present – individuals cannot become happier or more fulfilled by taking prescription drugs, as the advertisements suggest.

For the purposes of this book, medicalization is used as a platform for explaining how pharmaceutical advertisements decontextualize popular conceptions of health, ultimately reducing what it means to be healthy as becoming equated with previous, continued representations of medical science and/ or pharmaceutical drugs as forms of cultural authority. A more nuanced interpretation of this phenomenon can be explained via the theoretical foundation and social process of pharmaceuticalization.

PHARMACEUTICALIZATION

The theory of pharmaceuticalization has been present in sociology research for more than 20 years, yet recent work by scholars has allowed for explication of the term, referring also to the "pharmaceutical person," and the "pharmaceutical imagination" (Abraham 2009; Fox and Ward 2009; Marshall 2009; Martin 2006). Pharmaceuticalization explores society's over-reliance or dependence on drugs (Williams, Gabe, and Davis 2008). Pharmaceuticalization specifically addresses the ways in which pharmaceuticals have become woven into aspects of society, making the industry seem commonplace and the only option a consumer has when seeking information about their health. DTCA has been named as a crucial component of pharmaceuticalization, as the pharmaceutical industry uses these advertisements as a vehicle to obtain direct contact with the public. DTCA extends the relationship of prescription drug companies, physicians, and consumers in a very particular way that enhances the independent relationship between the consumer and the drug company (Conrad and Leiter 2004). As consumers are exposed to more pharmaceutical advertisements, they become more well-versed in brand names and celebratory depictions of medications rather than becoming educated on specific forms of illness or disease and alternative non-pharmaceutical options, ultimately meaning that patients are being trained by the media to consume more prescription drugs rather than being provided with the information necessary to make informed health care decisions.

Although both processes assume similar criteria, pharmaceuticalization cannot be completely subsumed under medicalization. Theorists have adapted a teleological approach to pharmaceuticalization, focusing mainly on the expansion and increase of prescription drugs throughout society (Clarke et al. 2003). Pharmaceuticalization can grow without the expansion of medicalization, as the pharmaceutical industry has come under fire for establishing specific medical conditions that warrant the use of their products – thus, transforming non-medical problems into medical ones (Abraham 2010). This growing presence of pharmaceuticals in society is referred to as a form of biomedicalism. The biomedicalism thesis states that a growth in prescription drugs can be attributed to the ability of progressive medicine to discover solutions for new or established illnesses (Conrad and Leiter 2008; Rose 2007). Pharmaceuticalization posits that this biomedicalism is taking place alongside an ideology of consumerism that characterizes advertising as being the driving force behind the cultural demand for prescription drugs (Applbaum 2006; Conrad 2007; Fox and Ward 2009; Marshall 2009; Rose 2007; Williams et al. 2009). Abraham (2010) has argued that pharmaceuticalization be framed using five explanatory factors, which are "mutually interactive but competing": biomedicalism (drug research, development, and innovation); medicalization; industry drug promotion and marketing; consumerism; and the ideology or policy of the regulatory state. As described in this chapter, the demand for prescription drugs is apparent, as the pharmaceutical industry is one of the most financially lucrative in the United States. Commodity fetishism can be used to demonstrate how this rise in consumerism permits the facets of pharmaceuticalization to not only increase in presence, but to become more seamlessly present in society.

"PHARMACEUTICAL FETISHISM" AND PSEUDO-INDIVIDUALITY/AUTONOMY FEATURED IN DTCA

The culmination of medicalization, pharmaceuticalization, and commodity fetishism can be used to explicate how processes of "pharmaceutical fetishism" are present in advertising culture. As sociological research has already established the relationships between consumerism and increased instances of medicalization and pharmaceuticalization, this book seeks to coin the term "pharmaceutical fetishism," related to the Marxian concept of "commodity fetishism."

By utilizing the theories of medicalization, pharmaceuticalization, and commodity fetishism, I am seeking to use this book as an opportunity to coin and define "pharmaceutical fetishism" as the commodification of brand-name pharmaceutical drugs, which, via advertising and promotional cultures, ignore large-scale production and for-profit motives of "big pharma" while simultaneously reiterating a brand discourse that offers individuals additionally constructed meanings and discourse which promote: medicine as a cultural authority in health care and prescription drugs as having the capability to solve individual problems beyond those for which a medicine is scientifically intended. The concept of pharmaceutical fetishism relies upon the forms of pseudo-autonomy presented to consumers, namely through DTC advertisements.

Recall the earlier discussions of pseudo-individuality, commodity fetishism, and advertising as magic. These arguments can be applied specifically to DTC advertisements to develop the concept of "pharmaceutical fetishism." This book is coining pharmaceutical fetishism as the ability of DTC advertisements to present consumers with romanticized portrayals regarding what benefits a prescription drug can offer and ignoring other treatment options. Rather than relying merely on the medical benefits associated with a drug designed to treat a target condition, the industry of DTCA has permitted these commercials to include "additional benefits," usually by relying on the use of emotional appeals or presentations of scenarios of those in the ads who have used the drugs. This means that the culture of prescription drugs is being reproduced, potentially suggesting to consumers that they can obtain positive attributes beyond what can be corrected in the body – for example, advertisements for antidepressants often feature all relationships as significantly improving and seeming "perfect" as a result of consuming a medication, but this is a veiled representation of a serious mental health condition and the social challenges that come along with it. In order to benefit capitalistic endeavors, the culture of pharmaceuticals has evolved into one that promises much more than it can realistically deliver for consumers. As Rose (2007) has suggested, DTCA may be an aspect of medicalization and pharmaceuticalization that creates false needs for consumers.

Furthermore, false claims are presented to consumers that lead them to believe that pharmaceuticals can meet individual needs and desires. This can be described as a form of ideological appropriation, as the industry that exists to expand understandings of health is the very industry that creates false needs in a consumer-driven market (Abraham 2010). Pharmaceutical fetishism will be an important underpinning for the examination of this book's sample, allowing empirical data to be viewed through a more critical lens.

HOW A MIXED-METHODS APPROACH PROVIDES AN EMPIRICAL FOUNDATION FOR DEEPER CRITICAL CONSIDERATIONS

Critical Advertising Studies as a subfield is about much more than textually analyzing advertisements, which itself is extremely important. Beyond deconstructing advertisements and their potential implications, this subfield aims to explain the larger context of an industry that is based on capital and mass production. By offering both a message-oriented analysis and industry structural analysis of the field, this framework attempts to understand mass culture and its impact on society. This allows researchers to further explicate the system of ideology that exists within promotional culture – one which encompasses the beliefs, values, and aspirations of an audience to ultimately persuade them into performing a behavior of purchasing (Turow and McAllister 2009). Dissecting advertisements and the advertising industry, both culturally and financially, is at the root of Critical Advertising Studies, a field which aims to respond to the consistently changing structures of mass communications and the media.

By relying on the aforementioned roots in Critical Advertising Studies, this book seeks to look at issues of representation and how these representations lend to an ideology of consumerism that celebrates the commodification of what was historically intended to be an effort to increase the health of human beings. Instead, pharmaceutical advertisements serve as a form of promotion for capitalism, ultimately placing a profit-making opportunity above elements of patient education and health initiatives. It is my intent to flesh out the meaning-making practices and strategies of prescription drug advertisements; by describing the "promises" these advertisements may offer patients, (i.e. happiness, success, love), and how the educational forms for which these promotions were originally intended may not exist or may not be as recognizable by consumers can be further discussed.

As Conrad (2007) has written, one of the primary drivers of medicalization and pharmaceuticalization has been an increase in consumerism, for which the pharmaceutical industry offers a telling example. Medicalization theorist John Abraham has even called for a critical study of this industry, but one that also utilizes "empirical realism" in order to fully show the problematic nature of pharmaceuticals within the context of this consumerist-driven paradigm (Abraham 2010). Of the limited research done on broadcast versions of DTC advertisements, content analysis is a popular method utilized. As many assumptions are made concerning media content, content analysis permits researchers to see whether specific content is actually present. Additionally, content analysis permits replicable and valid inferences to be drawn from texts. In order to more qualitatively and critically analyze the content of DTC advertisements, this book will perform a content analysis to provide an empirical foundation for deeper inquiry. Upon conducting quantitative research, textual analysis relying on principles of aforementioned Critical Advertising Studies aids in addressing the shortcomings of content analysis as a quantitative research method, as textual analysis will permit for more detailed descriptions of the implications regarding ultimate findings. By combining data across the paradigms of quantitative and qualitative research, this book can flesh out a richer understanding of the phenomena that extends how the processes of pharmaceutical fetishism operate. As pharmaceutical fetishism has many different aspects to consider, it is necessary to utilize all approaches in an effort to provide a comprehensive, holistic understanding of DTCA.

Holsti's (1969) literature emphasizes a particular way of approaching a mixed-method study in order to achieve the most holistic study, and these guidelines are followed in this book. As Holsti (1969) recommends, manifest content is analyzed, making inferences by objectively and systematically identifying specified characteristics of messages. Upon taking these steps via a quantitative content analysis, inferences about the results found are discussed (either regarding the specific messages analyzed or the potential effects of such messages), leading to a more critical and qualitative framework (Jordan et al. 2009).

By reviewing the content of the most broadcasted prescription drug advertisements of a particular time period, we can gain a broader understanding of how health is being framed by the drug industry. Additionally, the concept of pharmaceutical fetishism in association with these advertisements is useful in understanding how our society understands the process of seeking medical treatment and what it means to be healthy, ultimately leading consumers to believe that prescription drugs can offer personal and emotional benefits in addition to acting as remedies for the human body.

It is necessary to examine the ideological nature of these advertisements, which includes their primary and secondary discourses. The primary discourse of an advertisement looks at specific qualities of an advertised product, whereas secondary discourses investigate the social relationships that are embedded within the advertisements (O'Barr 1994). To summarize, by focusing a portion of this book on the replication on quantitative inquiry in order to obtain an empirical foundation, an exploration of how medicalization, pharmaceuticalization, and pharmaceutical fetishism are present within the current structure of DTCA can be best described.

Chapter 3

An Analysis of Primetime Television Featuring DTCA

The previous chapter discussed the critical orientation of this book while addressing the importance of a mixed-methods approach in deconstructing advertisements that have an empirical foundation. The commercialized nature of the prescription drug industry permits a domain (health) that we normally would not associate with being primarily about commodification or capital to be seen as acceptably commercial. For patients, traditional understandings label the most important relationship as that between them and their doctor, one that relies upon communication, confidentiality, and mutual trust. Through promotional culture, specifically advertising, the pharmaceutical industry has inserted itself into this dyadic relationship, creating an environment that re-defines patients as consumers. The relationship of the pharmaceutical industry to a patient should be fiduciary in nature, with a goal of protecting the health and education of the patient; instead, pharmaceutical advertisements change the landscape of this relationship into one that privileges selling products above all else.

Analyzing the specific symbols and appeals used in these advertisements through content analysis, this chapter addresses the potential misrepresentation of health risks and consequences associated with consuming prescriptions, providing a foundation for a more critical analysis to be conducted in chapter five. Chapter two pointed out that most DTC advertisement content analyses do not study television commercials, while those that do are somewhat dated (as of 2016), and are limited to variables that focus on the "rational vs. emotional appeal" framework. Updating common themes seen in prescription advertisements is useful for extending and adding to Frosch et al.'s (2007) original research in an effort to develop appropriate empirical foundations for deconstructing pharmaceutical and health care advertisements in the United States. This chapter provides the method, outline, and results of a quantitative content analysis conducted using a sample of DTC advertisements from primetime television broadcasting in 2010, in an effort to address the educational and/or informational aspects of DTCA. As will be shown, many of Frosch et al.'s results were found to still be characteristic of broadcast DTC advertisements, with some characteristics even more prominent than in the original study. Similar to the findings of Frosch et al., this concludes that DTC advertisements undermine their informational function by emphasizing overwhelmingly positive outcomes of drug use and discouraging serious considerations of risk factors and other treatment options.

PREVIOUS DTCA RESEARCH UTILIZING CONTENT ANALYSES

As reviewed earlier, a significant debate with DTCA revolves around the pharmaceutical industry's intentions. Proponents of DTCA claim that ads have the ability to educate consumers on various health conditions, leaving them empowered in seeking treatment options (Desselle and Aparasu 2000; Holmer 1999; Holmer 2002). Opponents of DTCA are critical of advertisements' abilities to mislead consumers (especially in terms of medication efficacy and the downplaying of risk), potentially causing them to ask their physicians for drugs they may not need, or that may be more expensive and physically intrusive than other lifestyle changes or treatment options (Hollon 1999; Mintzes 2002). To briefly return to earlier points, two paradigms exist in looking at the regulation of DTC advertisements. The first involves the FDA's regulatory role in ensuring that pharmaceutical advertisements are clearly and easily understood, putting patients in the position to be more fully informed about their medication options. A second paradigm exists, whereby these advertisements are seen as a mechanism for turning medications into commodities, being seen as a strong force in the capitalist market as opposed to being used for the originally intended purpose: to help maintain or improve the health of individuals. It is important to note that these two paradigms may be seen as mutually exclusive upon further review of the literature available. The research presented here suggests that "information" and "persuasion" discussed in research studies may not, in fact, be mutually exclusive.

The debate over DTC advertisements on television is complicated because of the mix of information versus influence, meaning that while these commercials may inform consumers of a prescription drug and its properties, they may also act as a form of influence for consumers to believe they need the product even if this may not be the case. Critics argue that the persuasive function is highlighted in these advertisements, while the informative aspects are marginalized in less identifiable formats. Main, Argo, and Huhman's

2004 content analysis of broadcast DTC advertisements focused on the proportion of rational (informative) versus emotional (persuasive) appeals (Main, Argo, and Huhman 2004). This study found that emotional appeals were used far more than informative appeals, with one third of the advertisements relying on informative techniques, and two thirds of the advertisements using persuasive techniques. Perhaps one of the most influential research studies to focus on broadcast versions of DTC advertisements was published in 2007 by Frosch et al., a study that, according to Google Scholar in 2016, has been cited nearly 200 times.

Frosch et al.'s study analyzed the content of pharmaceutical advertisements, using a sample of evening news and primetime programming from 2004 to determine content of the ads, specifically looking to see whether pharmaceutical companies were educating patients on target conditions and not simply emphasizing the medication itself. Advertisements were coded for factual claims made about a target condition, attempts made at appealing to consumers, and how medication and lifestyle behaviors were portrayed in the lives of advertisement characters. The random sample featured 103 advertisements comprising 31 unique prescription medications

Table 3.1   Prescription Drug Advertisements Captured in Frosch et al. (2007) Sample

Brand Name	Manufacturer	Advertised Indication
Actonel	Proctor & Gamble	Osteoporosis
Allegra	Aventis	Allergies
Ambien	Sanofi-Synthelabo	Insomnia
Celebrex	Pfizer	Osteoarthritis, rheumatoid arthritis
Cialis	Lilly ICOS	Erectile dysfunction
Crestor	AstraZeneca	Hypercholesterolemia
Detrol LA	Pfizer	Overactive bladder
Enbrel	Immunex	Rheumatoid arthritis
Fosamax	Merck	Osteoporosis
Lamisil	Novartis	Onychomycosis
Levitra	Bayer	Erectile dysfunction
Lipitor	Pfizer	Hypercholesterolemia
Nexium	AstraZeneca	Gastroesophageal reflux disease
Diovan	Novartis	Hypertension
Diovan HCT	Novartis	Hypertension
Lotrel	Novartis	Hypertension
Plavix	Bristol-Myers Squibb	Acute coronary syndrome
Prevacid	TAP	Gastroesophageal reflux disease
Procrit	Amgen	Chemotherapy-related anemia
Singulair	Merck	Allergies
Valtrex	GlaxoSmithKline	Genital herpes
Zelnorm	Novartis	Irritable bowel syndrome with constipation
Zocor	Merck	Hypercholesterolemia
Zoloft	Pfizer	Depression, social anxiety disorder

Note: Table created by Janelle Applequist.

This study can be considered one of the most important in DTCA to date as it is one of the first to analyze such a large sample of broadcast advertisements, which combine visual imagery, music, spoken words, and more intricate stories in an effort to appeal to more consumers. This was the first DTC advertisement study to systematically analyze what television advertisements claim about health conditions, how these advertisements attempt to appeal to consumers, and how they portray the role of lifestyle behaviors and medication in achieving good health (Frosch et al. 2007). The study found that the majority of prescription drug advertisements from their sample (82%) made factual claims about the condition a drug was designed to treat, yet few described condition causes (26%), risk factors for a condition (26%), or prevalence (25%). The study also found that emotional appeals were nearly universal (95%), with the ability to regain control as a result of taking the medication (85%) as a major theme.

Although Frosch et al.'s (2007) study used broadcast versions of advertisements, and included a large number of variables, health communication scholarship aiming to contextualize DTCA according to patient understandings would benefit from an updated study with a more recent sample to see how these advertisements have remained the same and/or changed, and also a more descriptive analysis of the results, with critical-cultural methodologies describing how pharmaceutical advertisements may be portraying characters as losing control over their social and emotional selves, while minimizing efforts on health conditions and maximizing persuasive appeals in efforts to increase profits. If these advertisements are selling products that can not only interfere with one's health, but can introduce an individual to a product that could potentially prove deadly, or at the least can undermine non-pharmaceutical treatment or lifestyle options, then it is crucial that research begin to more descriptively address how patients are being framed, and how conceptions of health care have become commodified, in an effort to offer solutions for increased patient education initiatives. To best address a more critical analysis of DTC advertisements, it is first necessary to obtain an empirical, quantitative foundation from which inferences can be made. This chapter quantitatively replicates previous research on DTC advertisements, providing a framework for more qualitative analyses to be conducted in chapters five and six.

The study presented in this chapter provides an extension to Frosch et al.'s research, using a more current sample of advertisements from 2010 in order to replicate and update the literature. The focus of this chapter is on the educational or informative aspects of DTC advertisements, which aligns with previous quantitative approaches to DTCA. Three categories were added to the replication of Frosch et al.'s (2007) work (animation, financing offers, and the use of before and after portrayals associated with consuming a prescription drug), as these were seen as emergent themes throughout the data. In addition to the finding that pharmaceutical advertisements are continuing to portray characters as losing control over their social and emotional selves, while minimizing educational efforts on health conditions and maximizing persuasive appeals in order to sell more prescriptions, suggesting that a more critical view of the content of prescription advertisements is necessary.

THEORETICAL FOUNDATIONS FOR ARGUMENTS

Other literatures are useful in developing arguments and making analytical connections for this book. One such literature, for example, is derived from standard media effects work. Two particular theories can be used to provide a solid framework for analyzing the results and that can complement a more critical orientation that will be used in the following chapters.

In previous health communication research utilizing content analyses, two theoretical perspectives are often used when making the assumption that media content has an effect on health behaviors: Gerbner's Cultivation Theory and Bandura's Social Cognitive Theory (Manganello and Fishbein 2009). Cultivation Theory posits that through socialization, individuals who consume media more frequently are more likely to view the world in a way that is consistent with that media; thus, content analysis can assess the amount of a particular type of content on television to understand the extent to which viewers are exposed to a particular belief system (Comstock, Lloyd-Jones, and Rubinstein 1972). Social Cognitive Theory looks at specific elements of media portrayals, assuming that portrayals of certain types of behavior will impact the behavior of the audience when paired with particular characteristics (i.e. if the media's portrayal of a behavior results in reward or punishment) (Bandura 2002). Additionally, Social Cognitive Theory is useful in content analysis, as it permits the researcher to investigate the concept of modeling, meaning that those who view a role model or actor engaging in a positively reinforced behavior may be more likely to engage in the behavior themselves (Bandura 2002). While Frosch et al. did not use these theoretical foundations in their research, previous quantitative research on DTCA has relied on these approaches in order to describe how these advertisements serve as forms of observational learning for health care. This means that, the more individuals are exposed to DTC advertisements, the more they may begin to embrace the world and behavioral incentives that DTCA portrays: so the more they may feel that they are in need of a particular prescription – or prescriptions generally – in order to remedy a health ailment they are experiencing, as opposed to seeking different treatment options such as lifestyle changes (Bergner et al.

2013; Hyojin and Chunsik 2012). Additionally, these theories have been used in DTCA research to show that individuals perceive more rewards being present after viewing an advertisement than simply gaining benefits for a health condition; this means that individuals respond positively to the ways in which drug advertisements are consistent with, and build on, socially constructed realities (Welch Cline and Young 2004).

As this book is an extension of the previously developed coding categories of Frosch et al. (2007), it is an attempt to replicate and update the DTCA literature with more current data in order to show if (and if so, how) DTC advertisements remained the same and/or changed since the evaluation of advertisements aired in 2004. By addressing any similarities or changes, we can better understand the content of DTCA. Once a strong foundation is provided regarding the content of these advertisements, media effects research can then investigate whether these advertisements impact consumer prescription drug choices, how patients feel prescription drug benefits and consequences compare to the representations shown in these advertisements, and whether pharmaceutical companies are compliant with the rules and regulations put in place by the FDA. Second, this work considers what types of characters are portrayed in pharmaceutical advertisements. This inquiry is useful in that it can shed light on the ways in which the pharmaceutical industry not only views consumers (or at least how the industry wants the consumers to view themselves), but in what ways niche markets are being targeted using specific representations and appeals. Finally, this is an attempt to describe how DTCA positions the role of medication in the lives of consumers. Most importantly, this book argues for an empirical, research-oriented approach to the subject in order to then open up important dialogue considering pharmaceutical culture in the United States.

Regarding the empirically oriented approach mentioned, content analysis can be used for a wide range of research objectives, including (but not limited to) describing the substance of characteristics in message content; describing form characteristics of message content; making inferences regarding the producers of content; making inferences regarding the audiences of content; and determining the effects of content on an audience (Berelson 1952). More concisely, Carney (1971) indicates that three uses for this method include describing, testing hypotheses, and facilitating inferences. Neuendorf (2002) has been credited with a six-part definition of content analysis that captures the method's flexibility while highlighting the necessity for proper study design and execution on part of the researcher. First, content analysis relies on the scientific method, meaning that is focuses on objectivity, a priori design, measurement, representation, and interpretation (Neuendorf 2002). An a priori design is one that makes all decisions on variables, their measurement, and coding rules before any observations begin in the research.

Second, content analysis relies on a message or group of messages that is used as the unit of analysis, unit of data collection, or in some cases, both. Third, content analysis is quantitative, meaning that the researcher's goal should be to produce counts of categories and measurements assigned to specific variables. As Gray and Densten (1998) describe, quantitative and qualitative research may be used as different methodologies for examining the same research problem, where multi-methodological triangulation "strengthens a researcher's claims for validity of the conclusions drawn where mutual confirmation of results can be demonstrated" (Gray and Densten 1998, 420). While the focus of this chapter is on the quantitative method of content analysis, it is important to note that triangulation can lead to the most comprehensive form of research if conducted properly, justifying the use of contrasting methods in the following chapter. Neuendorf's fourth aspect for the definition is that it summarizes themes chosen by the researcher, and the fifth element includes the method's applicability to all contexts (including interpersonal messages, organizational messages, and mass messages) (Neuendorf 2002).

Researchers have described two types of content: manifest and latent. The majority of content analysis research focuses on manifest content, meaning those elements which are physically present and countable (Gray and Densten 1998). Latent content includes that which may not be measured directly, but can be represented or measured by one or more indicators (Hair et al. 1998). Manifest content looks at the surface of a message, whereas latent content looks at the deeper structure by inferring from symbols used. Original conceptions of content analysis, such as that of Berelson's (1952) description, emphasize the use of manifest content only, but research now promotes the use of latent constructs as a way of integrating quantitative and qualitative analyses (Gray and Densten 1998).

Although this book is referencing television commercials from 2010, using DTC advertisements from 2010 is justifiable for two reasons. First, there have been no significant amendments to the Food and Drug Administration's (FDA) requirements or policies for pharmaceutical companies broadcasting product advertisements or changes proposed by the FCC for the advertisement of pharmaceutical drugs from 2010 to the time of this writing (2014). Second, Frosch et al. (2007) relied on a sample that was three years old as well, as the advertisements were readily available. This dataset was collected as part of a previous study conducted by another researcher on major environmentalism and green washing. The dataset was initially coded by the original researcher according to types of advertisements, including a category of pharmaceuticals. However, for this current study, the entire dataset was re-analyzed and re-coded to comprehensively identify the DTC advertisements as well as to add several other additional variables. Data from the broadcasting networks (as opposed to the lower-rated cable networks) is appropriate for the lens of these arguments as major broadcasting networks still focus on breadth and more generalized audiences, whereas emphasizing smaller niche networks would provide a more targeted consumer demographic. Additionally, this book seeks to emphasize the medium which provides the most accessibility for individuals, and as not every individual in the United States has cable television, major networks provide a platform from which to draw the most generalizable results, achieving the highest ratings and serving the greatest variety of consumer types.

Frosch et al.'s (2007) study included ads from primetime programming and evening news programs of the four largest U.S. broadcast networks (ABC, CBS, NBC, and Fox). Programming for their research was recorded for four consecutive weeks through June and July in 2004, with a different channel randomly selected for each day, with each day of the week represented for each network. This dataset includes all advertisements aired for all days of primetime programming across the four major broadcast television networks (ABC, CBS, NBC, and Fox) from February 1 to May 2, 2010. Unlike the research of Frosch et al., all programming was recorded and accounted for. This equates to ninety days of primetime programming, or 12 weeks and one day of recordings. Commercials for DTC prescription drugs were coded only; over-the-counter medications were excluded. The total 984 hours of recording for this study included 805 DTC ads, most of them repeating airings of the same advertisements. Frosch et al.'s study captured 103 DTC advertisements comprising 31 unique product claim ads. The original study of Frosch et al. of 2004 advertisements also included "reminder" ads – abbreviated ads which give the drug's name but not elaborations of its use – but the current study only analyzed product claim ads, meaning pharmaceutical advertisements that explicitly named a drug and included product risks and sources for more information. For the purposes of this book, 36 unique advertisements for 25 different prescription drugs were collected. This recording captured television commercials for 6 of the 10 top-selling prescription drugs in 2010, and 9 of the 10 most advertised prescription drugs in 2010 (Herper 2011; Kantar Media 2011). The specific medications featured in this sample are shown in Table 3.2; with the number of times each ad aired during the collection period documented to show the repetitive nature of the pharmaceutical industry's marketing efforts.

The majority of the prescription drugs featured in the 2010 sample used for this study had staying power in terms of sales and advertising spending. Table 3.3 lists a random sample of five prescriptions that were featured in this sample and shows the sales and rank of each drug for each year since the sample collection period in order to show that drugs captured in this dataset have remained prominent in the pharmaceutical market.

Table 3.2   Prescription Drug Advertisements Captured in Current Dataset

Prescription Brand Name	Number of Times Ad Aired During Sample Period	Manufacturer	Advertised Indication	Number of Ad Versions Featured in Sample
Abilify	14	Bristol-Myers Squibb Co.	Depression	2
Advair	78	GlaxoSmithKline	Asthma, COPD (Chronic Obstructive Pulmonary Disease)	3
Avodart	25	GlaxoSmithKline	BPH (Benign Prostatic Hyperplasia)	1
Boniva	14	Roche Group	Osteoporosis	1
Cialis	52	Eli Lilly	Erectile dysfunction	2
Crestor	59	AstraZeneca	High cholesterol, Atherosclerosis	2
Cymbalta	43	Eli Lilly	Depression	1
Lipitor	45	Pfizer	High cholesterol, high triglycerides, stroke prevention, heart attack prevention	2
Lovaza	14	GlaxoSmithKline	High triglycerides	1
Lunesta	8	Dainippon Sumitomo Pharma. Co. Ltd.	Insomnia	1
Lyrica	39	Pfizer	Fibromyalgia	2
Nasonex	65	Merck	Seasonal and perennial allergies	1
Omnaris	47	Dainippon Sumitomo Pharma. Co. Ltd.	Seasonal and perennial allergies, allergic rhinitis	1
Plavix	48	Bristol-Myers Squibb Co.	Stroke prevention, heart attack prevention	2
Pristiq	42	Pfizer	Depression	1
Restasis	9	Allergan Inc.	Chronic dry eye	2
Seroquel XR	12	AstraZeneca	Bipolar depression, depression, schizophrenia	12
Simponi	14	Janseen Pharmaceuticals	Rheumatoid arthritis, psoriatic arthritis	1
Spiriva	7	Boehringer Ingelheim Inc.	Emphysema, chronic bronchitis, COPD	1
Symbicort	64	AstraZeneca	Asthma, chronic bronchitis, COPD	3
Toviaz	31	Pfizer	Overactive bladder	1
Trilipix	27	Abbott Laboratories	High cholesterol, high triglycerides	1
VESIcare	16	Astellas Pharma Inc.	Overactive bladder	1
Viagra	9	Pfizer	Erectile dysfunction	1
YAZ	23	Bayer	Contraceptive, PMDD (Premenstrual Dysphoric Disorder)	1

Note: Table created by Janelle Applequist.

Table 3.3 Profile of Drugs Advertised in Current Sample and Endurance in Market-place from 2010 to 2013

			2010	
Prescription	Manufacturer	Advertised Indication	U.S. Sales (in billions)	Rank in U.S. Sales of All Prescription Drugs
Abilify	Bristol-Myers Squibb Co.	Depression	$4.6	3
Advair	GlaxoSmithKline	Asthma, COPD	$4.7	4
Cialis	Eli Lilly	Erectile Dysfunction	$658 million	47
Cymbalta	Eli Lilly	Depression	$3.2	13
Lipitor	Pfizer	High triglycerides, stroke prevention, heart attack prevention	$7.2	1
			2011	
Abilify	Bristol-Myers Squibb Co.	Depression	$5.0	4
Advair	GlaxoSmithKline	Asthma, COPD	$4.5	5
Cialis	Eli Lilly	Erectile Dysfunction	$200 million	80
Cymbalta	Eli Lilly	Depression	$3.5	9
Lipitor	Pfizer	High triglycerides, stroke prevention, heart attack prevention	$9.6	1
			2012	
Abilify	Bristol-Myers Squibb Co.	Depression	$5.6	2
Advair	GlaxoSmithKline	Asthma, COPD	$4.6	4
Cialis	Eli Lilly	Erectile Dysfunction	$237 million	79
Cymbalta	Eli Lilly	Depression	$4.5	5
Lipitor	Pfizer	High triglycerides, stroke prevention, heart attack prevention	$579 million	20
			2013	
Abilify	Bristol-Myers Squibb Co.	Depression	$6.3	1
Advair	GlaxoSmithKline	Asthma, COPD	$5.0	6
Cialis	Eli Lilly	Erectile Dysfunction	$1.1	48
Cymbalta	Eli Lilly	Depression	$5.1	5
Lipitor	Pfizer	High triglycerides, stroke prevention, heart attack prevention	Not available – no longer listed as a top 100 profiting drug as Lipitor lost exclusivity rights in 2011 allowing generic versions to enter the market	Not available

Note: Table created by Janelle Applequist.

The emphasis of this content analysis is the replication of Frosch et al.'s previous study, which developed coding categories that focused on the educational or informative nature of DTC advertisements. Prior to replicating the original coding scheme, I added two categories for quantitative analysis that were apparent themes in the advertisements – offers for financing assistance and/or free trial versions of prescription drugs and the use of animation to inform consumers of a health condition or used as a medical model/diagram. As in Frosch et al.'s original study, previously developed coding categories for print ads were used to serve as the coding foundation for the current study (Bell, Wilkes, and Kravitz 2000; Main, Argo, and Huhmann 2004). Two coding categories from Frosch et al. were not considered. The first was "biological nature or mechanism of disease," as coders agreed that this category could be synonymous with "any factual information on a condition" being presented (these categories were combined). The second was "risk factors or cause of condition," which was also agreed to be synonymous with "any factual information on a condition" being present.

Seeing that proponents of DTCA claim that the advertisements serve as a form of public education, one central goal of this content analysis was to determine the frequency with which television advertisements made factual claims about conditions or diseases. Categories coded in Frosch et al.'s original study and used in this current study include (1) rational appeals – providing information about product use, features, or comparison with similar products; (2) positive emotional appeals – evoking favorable affect; (3) negative emotional appeals – evoking negative affect through emotions such as fear; (4) humor appeals; (5) fantasy appeals – depicting unrealistic or surreal scenes; (6) sex appeals – depicting intimate situations; (7) nostalgic appeals – using sepia-toned or black-and-white imagery (Main, Argo, and Huhmann 2004; Frosch et al. 2007).

A significant criterion applied to content analysis is the concept of reliability, or the "extent to which a measuring procedure yields the same results on repeated trials" (Carmines and Zeller 1979). Intercoder reliability is calculated for human coders used in content analysis research (also referred to as intercoder agreement) in order to discover how different judges assign the same rating to an object, using a method where objectivity and universality are prominent goals (Tinsley and Weiss 1975). Specifically, reliability is a way of measuring a study's stability, reproducibility, and accuracy (Krippendorff 2004). Without reliability, the findings of a study cannot be considered objective enough to be replicated and generalized among a larger sample. Although there is no consensus on a single best reliability index to use, many in content analysis literature have claimed that Cohen's kappa is supreme (Dewey 1983). In health communication research, Cohen's kappa is one of the most popular choices in calculating intercoder reliability (e.g. see Chmura

Kraemer, Periyakoil, and Noda 2002; Guggenmoos-Holzmann 1996; Thompson et al. 2003; Vach 2005).

Neuendorf (2002) reviewed the most popular reliability coefficients and determined a suggested set of guidelines for acceptable levels based on previous studies (particularly Banerjee et al. 1999; Ellis 1994; Frey, Botan, and Kreps 2000; Krippendorff 2004; Popping 1988; Riffe, Lacy, and Fico 2005). The analysis found that "coefficients of 0.90 or greater would be acceptable for all research studies, 0.80 or greater would be deemed acceptable in most situations, and below that, there exists disagreement" (Neurendorf 2002). Krippendorff (2004) recommends 0.80 or greater with the use of two or more coders, and other research has shown that 0.70 or above is acceptable for exploratory studies (Lombard, Snyder-Duch, and Campanella Bracken 2006).

Myself, one master's-level research assistant, and one bachelor's-level research assistant were trained for three hours each and coded all of the advertisements in this dataset independently. Statistical Package for the Social Sciences (SPSS) analysis of variance (ANOVA) statistics software was used to analyze this dataset and to check for intercoder reliability. "Very good" aggregate intercoder reliability was found for coding categories, as indicated by Cohen's kappa values ranging from 0.88–0.91 (Cohen 1960; Cohen 1968; Neurendorf 2002). For all cases ($n = 1,656$) and decisions ($n = 4,968$), the average pairwise agreement among the three coders was 95.0%, with the overall average kappa value being 0.89. Cohen's kappa accounts for chance agreement with the added benefit of accounting for differences in the distribution of values across categories for different coders (Cohen 1960; Cohen 1968).

It is also necessary to discuss the concept of validity, or the extent to which a measuring procedure represents an intended concept. First, focusing on the current chapter and its accompanying quantitative analysis, the coding schemes used in previous content analysis has been argued to be a legitimate mechanism to achieve a high level of construct validity, meaning that a measure correlates with other measures of the same construct (Brinberg and Kidder 1982). The coding in this chapter is an extension of previously used and tested coding categories, and therefore its measures have been previously established and replicated, making these coding categories, techniques, and subsequent findings valid. More specifically, using previously developed codebooks, and adding to definitions in cases where ambiguity may have been possible, the construct validity of this portion of the study is increased.

Additionally, from a broader perspective that considers the totality of this book, validity was cross-checked in multiple ways. Multiple methods, including the use of textual analysis to complement the content analysis, helped to ensure that the codebooks being used for this book were strengthening the overall argument rather than raising more questions. Triangulation confirmed that when all results are combined, a more robust picture of what is taking place is present, especially given the high level of agreement of the results across methods. Rather than achieve triangulation only through the use of multiple methods, this book also utilized multiple theoretical foundations to look at important questions needing answered; both the quantitative and qualitative results were consistent with the theoretical orientation offered in previous chapters. Finally, it is important that researchers detail their data collection and coding processes to ensure a higher level of validity, which was a goal throughout the writing of this book.

The specific coding categories and results for Frosch et al.'s study (2007) are shown in Table 3.4, with the coding categories used in this study and their respective results shown in Table 3.5.

Table 3.4   Proportion of Advertisements that Present Factual Claims, Appeals, Lifestyle, and Medication Themes from Frosch et al. (2007)

Categories of Content	Product Claim Ads (Weighted Percentages)
Factual Claims	
Any factual information (i.e. symptoms)	82.0
Biological nature or mechanism of disease	53.9
Risk factors or cause of condition	25.8
Prevalence of condition	24.7
Subpopulation at risk of the condition	7.9
Appeals	
Rational	100.0
Positive emotional	94.4
Negative emotional	75.3
Humor	36.0
Fantasy	22.5
Sex	4.5
Nostalgia	3.4
Lifestyle portrayals	
Condition interferes with healthy or recreational activities	30.3
Product enables healthy or recreational activities	56.2
Lifestyle change is alternative to product use	0.0
Lifestyle change is insufficient	21.3
Lifestyle change is adjunct to product	22.5
Medication Portrayals	
Loss of control caused by condition	67.4
Regaining control as a result of product use	88.8
Social approval as a result of product use	83.1
Distress caused by condition	53.9
Breakthrough	67.4
Endurance increased as a result of product use	12.4
Protection as a result of product use	11.2

Note: Table created by Janelle Applequist.

Table 3.5 Proportion of Advertisements that Present Factual Claims, Appeals, Lifestyle, and Medication Themes for Current Study

Categories of Content	Advertisements (Percentage Category Representation out of 36 Unique Advertisements)
Factual Claims	
Any factual information (i.e. symptoms)	72.2
Prevalence of condition	5.6
Subpopulation at risk of the condition	16.7
Before and After Portrayal	
Before and after portrayed	44.4
Only before portrayed	0.0
Only after portrayed	47.2
Animation	
Animated mascot used for product	13.9
Graphic used to explain condition	36.1
Graphic used to explain medication	25.0
Manufacturer logo present portion of ad	66.7
Manufacturer logo present entire ad	0.0
Medication logo present portion of ad	66.7
Medication logo present entire ad after being named	36.1
Finance	
Offer to help afford prescription	52.8
Offer to receive free trial version	36.1
Appeals	
Rational	100.0
Positive emotional	94.4
Negative emotional	41.7
Humor	5.6
Fantasy	30.6
Sex	8.3
Nostalgia	8.3
Lifestyle Portrayals	
Condition interferes with healthy or recreational activities	66.7
Product enables healthy or recreational activities	91.7
Lifestyle change is alternative to product use	0.0
Lifestyle change is insufficient	5.6
Lifestyle change is adjunct to product	19.4
Medication Portrayals	
Loss of control caused by condition	52.8
Regaining control as a result of product use	97.2
Social approval as a result of product use	58.3
Distress caused by condition	66.7
Breakthrough	41.7
Endurance increased as a result of product use	72.2
Protection as a result of product use	72.2

Note: Table created by Janelle Applequist.

In order to most accurately update the literature according to the structure of Frosch et al.'s original research, the following findings will be categorized and presented in the same order published in 2007. To briefly compare the drugs captured in each sample, see Tables 3.1 and 3.2. Four drugs were captured in both this dataset and Frosch et al.'s study, including Cialis, Crestor, Lipitor, and Plavix. Within the current dataset, 15 prescription drugs are included that were introduced to the market after Frosch et al.'s use of ads from 2004, showing a significant increase in the number of new pharmaceuticals being advertised to consumers. The prescription drugs featured in the current dataset that were released after 2004 include: Abilify, Boniva, Cymbalta, Lunesta, Lyrica, Nasonex, Omnaris, Pristiq, Seroquel XR, Simponi, Spiriva, Symbicort, Trilipix, Toviaz, Vesicare, and YAZ ("FDA approval history" 2014).

AD LENGTH, STORY STRUCTURE, AND INFORMATIVE CONTENT

The average ad length from Frosch et al.'s (2007) product claim ad sample was 51.8 seconds. Ads in Frosch et al.'s sample showed characters before and after taking the product in 44.7% of the ads, with a smaller amount (39.5%) showing characters only after taking the medication, and 7.9% showing characters only before taking the product. The average ad length for the current dataset (see Table 3.6) was 56.1 seconds, showing an apparent increase in the length of prescription drug advertisements over a six-year airing period (2004 compared to 2010); however, the current dataset did not include "reminder ads" that were used in Frosch et al.'s research, which may confound the conclusion that DTCAs have increased in length.

More than 44% of advertisements showed characters before and after taking a medication, which is similar to the results found by Frosch et al. This indicates a continuation of a strategy where patients are typically portrayed as having a negative experience prior to consuming a medication and a much more positive experience after consumption. Characters were only shown after taking a medication in 47.2% of advertisements. As this book seeks to see how the content of DTC advertisements has changed and/or remained the same since the use of Frosch et al.'s original sample, this finding shows an increase in the positive associations shown after consumption of a medication in pharmaceutical advertisements (39.5% in Frosch et al.'s sample versus 47.2% in the current dataset). This shows that, overwhelmingly, pharmaceutical advertisements feature a character after they have taken a drug; 44.4% feature characters before and after they have obtained a prescription, with 47.2% showing characters only after they have obtained

Table 3.6 DTC Advertisements in Current Sample: Overall Ad Length versus Side Effect Narration Length

Prescription Drug Advertisement	Advertised Indication	Total Length of Advertisement (minutes: seconds)	Side Effect Narration Length in Advertisement (minutes: seconds)
Abilify (version 1)	Depression	1:15	0:41
Advair (version 1)	Asthma, COPD (Chronic Obstructive Pulmonary Disease)	1:00	0:19
Advair (version 2)	Asthma, COPD	1:00	0:12
Advair (version 3)	Asthma, COPD	1:00	0:08
Avodart	BPH (Benign Prostatic Hyperplasia)	1:00	0:12
Boniva	Osteoporosis	1:00	0:19
Cialis (version 1)	Erectile Dysfunction	1:00	0:20
Cialis (version 2)	Erectile Dysfunction	1:00	0:20
Crestor (version 1)	High cholesterol, Atherosclerosis	1:00	0:10
Crestor (version 2)	High cholesterol, Atherosclerosis	1:00	0:15
Cymbalta	Depression	1:15	0:30
Lipitor (version 1)	High cholesterol, High triglycerides, Stroke prevention, Heart attack prevention	1:00	0:09
Lipitor (version 2)	High cholesterol, High triglycerides, Stroke prevention, Heart attack prevention	1:00	0:15
Lovaza	High triglycerides	1:00	0:19
Lunesta	Insomnia	1:00	0:28
Lyrica (version 1)	Fibromyalgia	1:00	0:26
Lyrica (version 2)	Fibromyalgia	1:00	0:26
Nasonex	Seasonal & perennial allergies	0:30	0:07
Omnaris	Seasonal & perennial allergies, Allergic rhinitis	0:30	0:02
Plavix (version 1)	Stroke & heart attack prevention	1:00	0:30
Plavix (version 2)	Stroke & heart attack prevention	1:00	0:30
Pristiq	Depression	1:15	0:30
Restasis (version 1)	Chronic dry eye	0:30	0:10
Restasis (version 2)	Chronic dry eye	0:30	0:10
Seroquel XR	Bipolar Depression, Schizophrenia, Bipolar Disorder, MDD (Major Depressive Disorder)	1:30	0:50

Prescription Drug Advertisement	Advertised Indication	Total Length of Advertisement (minutes: seconds)	Side Effect Narration Length in Advertisement (minutes: seconds)
Simponi	Rheumatoid arthritis, Psoriatic arthritis	1:00	0:30
Spiriva	Emphysema, Chronic Bronchitis, COPD	1:00	0:21
Symbicort (version 1)	Asthma, chronic bronchitis, COPD	1:00	0:20
Symbicort (version 2)	Asthma, chronic bronchitis, COPD	1:00	0:18
Symbicort (version 3)	Asthma, chronic bronchitis, COPD	1:00	0:18
Toviaz	Overactive bladder	1:00	0:14
Trilipix	High cholesterol & high triglycerides	1:00	0:22
Vesicare	Overactive bladder	1:00	0:19
Viagra	Erectile Dysfunction	1:00	0:21
YAZ	Contraceptive, PMDD (Premenstrual Dysphoric Disorder)	1:10	0:30

Note: Table created by Janelle Applequist.

it, meaning that 91.6% of ads show the intended benefits associated with taking a prescription drug. The situations often point to the positive emotional effects present as a result of having the medication, rather than educating the audience on particular aspects of a medical condition. No advertisements featured only the "before" in a character's life, and rather always featured the benefits associated with obtaining a medication. In the instances where "before and after" or "after" were featured, the advertisements relied on setting a scene that emphasized an individual as more positive, happy, and healthy as a result of having the product. Most importantly, the use of "before" and "after" in pharmaceutical advertising points to the increase in the industry's use of relying more on benefits than side effects, but also denotes and further solidifies the use of pharmaceutical fetishism in consumer culture (see Table 3.7).

In an in-depth interview study of patient interpretations of five popular prescription drug advertisements, researchers found that viewers of pharmaceutical ads negotiate their personal sense of motivation toward lifestyle changes and/or prescription drug uptake by comparing themselves to scenarios depicted in the ads to their lived experiences, showing how consumers self-identify with the portrayals (Frosch et al. 2011). Researchers also found that consumers judged the perceived credibility of an advertisement based on its ability to connect with their own lives, possibly showing how the intended

Table 3.7 Examples of "Before and After" Used in Current DTC Advertisement Dataset

Prescription & Advertised Indication	Central Character(s)	"Before" Depiction	"After" Depiction
Abilify, depression (ads 1 & 2)	Wife/mother, middle-aged, white	Wife/mother is shown feeling distressed and turned away from her husband and teenage daughter while ad narrator states, "Approximately 2 out of 3 people treated for depression still have unresolved symptoms." Husband is shown glancing over at his wife with a look of concern as his daughter is talking to him.	Wife/mother is outside on a small island by the water with her teenage daughter and husband laughing and talking. Wife/mother is walking in a hallway at work interacting with a coworker while smiling. Wife/mother is in the movie theater with a friend, then shown leaving movie theater laughing and smiling. Ad ends with wife/mother speaking directly to camera while smiling, "Adding Ability has made a difference for me."
Cymbalta, depression	Father, male, middle-aged, African American; Wife, older adult, white; Single woman, middle-aged, white	Father is shown at work, leaning against a wall, distressed and alone. Wife is shown sitting at kitchen table alone, looking worried. Single woman is shown standing in house by herself visibly concerned	Father is shown in his bedroom playing with his daughters, lifting one in the air and carrying one on his back while smiling and laughing. Wife is shown holding hands with husband while inside house, looking outside the front door window to sunshine and smiling. Single woman is shown opening the curtains while in her house and smiling, then shown reading a book alone outside in a peaceful setting on her front porch
Lunesta, insomnia	Single woman, middle-aged, white	Single woman is in bed, her bed transforms into a boxing ring. She is shown tossing and turning, unable to sleep. She appears frustrated.	A green animated butterfly enters the bedroom, touches the velvet ropes surrounding the "boxing ring," and the ropes disappear, leaving a bed. The butterfly tucks in the woman, who is now asleep. The woman is shown in the mirror the next morning smiling and getting ready for her day.

| Viagra, Erectile Dysfunction | Older adult, male, African American | Male is shown in various situations, (in front of mirror, getting dressed, etc.) "practicing" alone and rehearsing how he would like to talk to his doctor about his sexual problems. Each "rehearsal" shows him nervous and apprehensive about the conversation, visibly distressed. | The male is shown talking to his doctor, and immediately after being handed a prescription for Viagra, he appears happy and energized. He leaves the doctor's office confidently, walking on the sidewalk smiling. He purchases flowers (assumed to be for a sexual partner) and happily walks away. |
| YAZ, contraceptive, PMDD | Single younger adult 1, female, white
Single younger adult 2, female, white
Single younger adult 3, female, white
Single younger adult 4, female, Asian | No characters are depicted in "before" setting, "after" is only scenario shown | Single younger adult 1 is sitting in the back of a cab, smiling directly at the camera. She leans forward into the camera, smiles, and playfully runs her hands through her hair. She is later shown in an art gallery with a friend laughing and smiling.
Single younger adult female 2 is fully clothed, shown laying in a bubble bath with her clothing still on, laughing at the camera.
Single younger adult female 3 is shown painting her walls bright orange. She looks over at the camera and smiles.
Single younger adult 4 is shown cutting her own hair and she does so in a playful way (not carefully). She cuts her own bangs and smiles at the camera. |

Source: Bayer 2010; Bristol-Myers Squibb Co. 2010c & 2010d; Dainippon Sumitomo Pharma. Co. Ltd. 2010; Eli Lilly 2010a; Pfizer 2010d).
Note: Table created by Janelle Applequist.

physical, and extended emotional/personal, benefits of a drug in an advertisement may lead viewers to believe more in the product and its effectiveness (Frosch et al. 2011). Table 3.7 provides five examples from this dataset which feature "before" and "after" depictions as presented to viewers, signifying how pharmaceutical fetishism celebrates the drug industry while offering patients additional benefits for their lifestyles aside from the medical reasons for which a prescription drug would be prescribed.

In accordance with FDA regulations, every product claim advertisement in this study provided major risk and side-effect information, and in all cases, this information was always provided in the latter part of the advertisement, which was true for Frosch et al.'s (2007) study as well. An interesting finding by Frosch et al. was that side-effect information was always featured in the second half of an advertisement, but in all cases, the final frames were not devoted to side effects, but rather to branding, logo placement, and further promotional messages, perhaps to end the advertisement on a "stronger" note. As was found in Frosch et al.'s original study, each advertisement in the current study complied with FDA regulations in terms of providing risk information, yet each advertisement featured a promotional message after these side effects to end the spot in a seemingly more positive way.

Frosch et al.'s study did not address the amount of time each DTC advertisement spent on narrating side effects, but the current research coded this information in an effort to show the advertising's acknowledge of the danger and risk associated with consuming pharmaceutical drugs (see Table 3.6). Additionally, providing this information sheds light on the significance of broadcast versions of these advertisements, as side effects are presented as voice-overs while at the same time consumers are shown multiple modalities – characters interacting, music being played, text being presented on the screen, etc. – all which may increase the likelihood that consumers do not, in fact, give their full attention to listening to the possible risks associated with taking these medications. The average length of total ad time for this dataset was 0:56 (seconds), with the average length of time attributed to disclaimers and narration of side effects being 0:25, nearly half the time of the average ad length. Overall, antidepressant advertisements generally took the most time to narrate possible side effects and risk information, with the average length of disclaimer and side effect narration in antidepressant advertisements being 0:30. For example, this dataset featured two versions of an advertisement for Abilify, a prescription that is meant to be added to an already-existing antidepressant regimen. Both advertisements last for 1:15 (minutes, seconds), with 0:41 (seconds) in each devoted to the listing of side effects and risk information. A notable finding related to the narration of side effect information is that 93.2% of this dataset featured the explanation of risks/side effects as the character being shown was simultaneously presenting the "after" of medication consumption. Consumers are being sent mixed messages – as they are being informed of potential risk factors associated with a particular prescription drug while at the same time they are shown characters that receive only positive attributes associated with the medication. In an advertisement for Simponi, a self-injectable prescription used for rheumatoid arthritis pain, stiffness, and swelling, the beginning of the storyline features no display of characters, only relying on shots of office desks and personal calendars with notes reading "out for a month," "gone for the month," and "bye," as the narration describes how these individuals are gone not because of their pain, but because they now have the ability to be more active thanks to the prescription (Janssen Pharmaceuticals 2010). The ad lasts for 1:00, with 0:30 devoted to side effects and risk factors, yet, three separate characters with distinct storylines appear as the voiceover begins. One woman is shown standing while watching her kids ride a carousel, a couple is laying on the beach and playfully jumps up to take a walk while watching the sunset, and a third character is shown shopping for shoes and eating lunch with a friend as she is carrying a shopping bag prominently featuring the Simponi logo. As these characters' storylines are being shown and developed during the 0:30 period, the voiceover explains that:

> Simponi is a prescription medicine. Simponi can lower your ability to fight infections. There are reports of serious infections caused by bacteria, fungi, or viruses that have spread throughout the body, including tuberculosis (TB) and histoplasmosis. Some of these infections have been fatal. Your doctor will test you for TB before starting Simponi and will monitor you for signs of TB during treatment. Tell your doctor if you have been in close contact with people with TB. Tell your doctor if you have been in a region (such as the Ohio and Mississippi River Valleys and the Southwest) where certain fungal infections like histoplasmosis or coccidioidomycosis are common. You should not start Simponi if you have any kind of infection. Tell your doctor if you are prone to or have a history of infections or have diabetes, HIV or a weak immune system. You should also tell your doctor if you are currently being treated for an infection or if you have or develop any signs of an infection such as: fever, sweat, or chills; muscle aches; cough; shortness of breath; blood in phlegm; weight loss; warm, red, or painful skin or sores on your body; diarrhea or stomach pain; burning when you urinate or urinating more than normal; or feeling very tired (Janssen Pharmaceuticals 2010).

The relationship of narrative development to the simultaneous narration of side effects and important warnings is also illustrated by Lunesta, a drug with especially alarming disclaimers. Described for insomnia and difficulty sleeping, Lunesta advertises itself as "being different" to other sleep aides, featuring a woman in bed late at night, tossing and turning, as boxing match bells ring and the narrator explains "If you've already taken a sleep aide, and you're still fighting to sleep in the middle of the night, why would you go one more

round using it? You don't need a re-match, but a re-think – with Lunesta"
(Dainippon Sumitomo Pharma. Co. Ltd. 2010). After introducing Lunesta, the
remaining 0:27 of the advertisement are devoted to the narrated side effects:

> When taking Lunesta, don't drive or operate machinery until you feel fully
> awake. Walking, eating, driving, or engaging in other activities while asleep
> without remembering it the next day have been reported. Abnormal behaviors
> may include: aggressiveness, agitation, hallucinations, or confusion. In depressed
> patients, worsening of depression, including risk of suicide, may occur. Alcohol
> may increase these risks. Allergic reactions such as tongue or throat swelling occur
> rarely and may be fatal. Side effects may include: unpleasant taste, headache, diz-
> ziness, and morning drowsiness (Dainippon Sumitomo Pharma. Co. Ltd. 2010).

As the voiceover explains that driving while asleep without remembering
these events the next day, the character is shown finally at peace, as she has
taken Lunesta and has the ability to fall asleep. The final 4 seconds of the
advertisement show the character waking up the following morning, in a
bright, cheerful, and serene setting, as if she is ready to take on the world.

Animation

Nearly 14% of the sample featured an animated mascot for a prescription.
Not only do these animations serve to perhaps minimize the seriousness associated with a medical condition, but they act as a means of brand association
for consumers. Research has shown that in order for brand or logo repetition in
broadcast advertisements to be effective, consumers must first have familiarity with the product being introduced (Campbell and Keller 2003). As shown
in Table 3.5, during the approximate 12-week sample period, many of the
prescription drugs featured in this sample were aired repeatedly, showing that
it is highly possible that consumers have already developed familiarity with
these brand names due to their reach and prevalence on television. It is likely
that animated logos and mascots are used in these ads as a means of increasing brand awareness and recognition. For example, individuals may be able
to recall that Lunesta advertisements feature a neon butterfly, or that Nasonex
is promoted by an animated bumblebee voiced by actor Antonio Banderas
(Dainippon Sumitomo Pharma. Co. Ltd 2010; Merck 2010). Similarly to this
type of branding, medication and manufacturer logos were present in 66.7% of
advertisements, with medication logos on screen during entire advertisements
after initially being named 36.1% of the time. This often reinforced brand
names among coders, increasing their abilities to be able to recall specific
information about a drug (i.e. Lipitor's heart logo was at the top right-hand
corner of the screen during the entire advertisement) (Pfizer 2010c). Graphics

were used to explain conditions (36.1%) and medication properties (25.0%), also utilizing animated features to educate and attract consumers. Even given the possible health risks associated with consuming prescription drugs, the space of health care is not one that is immune to the infiltration of marketing and corporate presence into everyday life (Klein 2000). Not only are medication logos featured in every advertisement in this sample, but the corporate giant behind the drug being suggestively sold (i.e. Merck, Pfizer, Eli Lilly) are all present as well, again reinforcing the marketing goals of this industry.

FINANCING OFFERS AND FREE TRIAL VERSIONS

Nearly 53% of ads included an offer to help patients afford the medication, with 36.1% mentioning free trial versions available (see Table 3.5). Free trial versions were always framed as being available only by visiting the medication's website to "learn more" or talking with a physician to receive free samples. Samples are beneficial in that they can be given to patients immediately needing to begin a treatment regimen, and on the surface, they may seem like a good way for patients to reduce the overall cost of a brand-name prescription drug. Many pharmaceutical companies claim that free samples are put in place to help those patients who cannot afford high medication prices. However, a 2008 study found that less than one third of patients receiving free samples are low-income individuals, with those in the highest income categories being more likely to receive them (Vincent 2008). The data also found that those with continuous health insurance were more likely to receive samples from their doctors than those with no form of health insurance. Additional studies have shown that free samples may not end up saving patients money long-term. Patients given free samples save an average of $66 over a period of six months. Physicians that are provided free samples of brand-name drugs and subsequently give those samples to patients are more likely to prescribe those medications than physicians who do not receive samples from sales representatives (Symm et al. 2006). Patients receiving free samples upon viewing a DTC advertisement and requesting a trial version have been found to pay higher out-of-pocket costs overall because of the association with a brand name (Chimonas and Kassiser 2009). It is possible that what may seem a positive step by drug companies (helping patients alleviate costs) is simultaneously reinforcing that the pharmaceutical industry is acting as an intermediary between patients and their physicians, ultimately diminishing the confidentiality of this relationship.

While the multiple modalities being used are understandably over-stimulating for consumers who may be attempting to learn about a prescription drug, perhaps the most problematic nature of these advertisements are the side effects themselves, and the little attention that is given to the seriousness of the subject. If, in fact, pharmaceutical companies were trying to inform patients above all else rather than simply trying to sell a product, then it would make sense that every modality used during the side effect portion of an advertisement would reinforce the importance of that information and direct the consumer's attention to becoming more educated. For example, rather than the Lunesta advertisement showing the positive appeals associated with the character getting to have a comfortable, restful night's sleep, the advertisement could have replaced that imagery with a text listing of the side effects and risk information to accommodate visual learners. Instead, the recurring theme seen in the entire dataset features a prominent "switch" during each advertisement – the storyline becomes more developed, positive, and nuanced once the side effects narration begins, arguably taking the attention of consumers away from the educational information being described and pushing them toward connecting more emotionally with the story unfolding before them.

FACTUAL CLAIMS ABOUT THE TARGET CONDITION

An important category for analysis includes the presentation of information about a target condition in pharmaceutical advertisements. As discussed in chapter two, the greatest debate in pharmaceutical advertising regards whether the messages serve as forms of suggestive promotion or education for consumers. As the pharmaceutical industry continues to claim that these advertisements are in place to inform consumers about negative health conditions and ailments, with a possible remedy being offered (via the prescription), then it is vital that research analyzes whether DTCA is presenting factual information about the conditions that particular prescriptions are designed to treat.

The results of Frosch et al.'s (2007) study showed that more than half (53.9%) presented information on the biological nature or mechanism of a particular disease, yet only 25.8% of advertisements described risk factors or causes of the condition. Nearly 25% addressed the population prevalence of a condition, but among this group, only 25% gave specific information (e.g. "2 in 8 will develop…"). Only 7.9% of their sample identified subpopulations at risk for a particular condition.

As shown in Table 3.5, this book shows that most of the advertisements (72.2%) presented factual information on the condition the prescription was targeting, often in terms of defining the condition or its symptoms. There has been an increase in the educational components seen in pharmaceutical advertising on television. However, this dataset was coded as being "informative on a condition" if the condition was mentioned or the negative attributes of the condition were mentioned in any way. It is not known whether Frosch et al. operationalized this concept in this way. A subpopulation that would be at most risk for developing the condition was only identified 16.7% of the time, and while this is a small increase since Frosch et al.'s research, this number contradicts the claim that DTCA uniformly serves as a form of educating the public about health conditions that may affect them. Of the advertisements that did mention a specific population, the terms used in every instance were extremely vague (i.e. "men," "women," "older women"). While many health ailments or conditions requiring medication are most often seen in more specific populations, pharmaceutical companies are better served by presenting populations at risk in more vague terms – by casting a wider net, there exists a greater potential for more individuals to consider obtaining the product.

APPEALS

Frosch et al. (2007) found that nearly all (94.4%) of advertisements used positive emotional appeals which depicted how a character acted upon seemingly having obtained a drug, usually indicated via character happiness. Approximately 75% of advertisements relied on the use of negative emotional appeals, such as showing a character in a fearful or depressed state prior to using the product. Other emotions utilized included humor (36%), fantasy (22.5%), sex (4.5%), and nostalgia (3.4%).

Every advertisement in this dataset presented rational information (i.e. warnings); however, positive emotional tactics were overwhelmingly used (94.4%), remaining consistent with the original findings of Frosch et al. Positive emotional tactics refers to characters in advertisements expressing emotions such as happiness, fulfillment, or increased activity as a result of having the product. Negative emotions were used in 41.7% of the advertisements featured in this dataset, and all instances of negative emotions featured a character prior to having obtained a prescription. These negative emotions were used most often in regards to inability to participate in social activities as a result of the medical condition (i.e. antidepressant advertisements showed the character as visibly distressed, often not participating in the nuclear family activities happening as they had to watch from afar). The use of negative emotional appeals in this dataset (41.7%) is a significant decrease from Frosch et al.'s finding of 75.3%, highlighting how the pharmaceutical industry has decreased the use of "fear appeals" in their advertising, and, instead, increased the modeling of the pseudo-agency and proactivity discussed in chapter two. Rather than relying on the negative aspects associated with disease, pharmaceutical advertisements are now relying more on attempts to have consumers connect with only the beneficial aspects of consuming a particular medication, in turn, increasing the presence of pharmaceutical fetishism discussed earlier.

In the advertisement for the antidepressant Cymbalta, for example, positive emotions are used for 1:00 of the 1:15 total, with only 0:15 actually portraying a character as depressed or feeling down. Rather than informing consumers about depression, the advertisement allots most of the time (0:30) to the side effects associated with the medicine, and portrays a series of different individuals who it is assumed have taken Cymbalta, as these individuals do not appear to be depressed, but rather, are experiencing positive, social, and warm events with loved ones. One character is featured with her partner, as they are smiling, laughing, and kissing; another character is shown camping with his family while enjoying a campfire; a young woman is shown sitting alone outside while reading a book; and a father is shown playing with his young daughter in his home (Eli Lilly 2010a). While these portrayals all convey positive emotions, it is interesting to note that, once again, the advertisement uses the time while these depictions are shown to describe the following, sending a very mixed message to consumers:

> Cymbalta is a prescription medication that treats many symptoms of depression. Tell your doctor right away if your depression worsens or if you have unusual changes in behavior or thoughts of suicide [voiceover occurs as a young woman is shown looking out the window of her home and smiling]. Antidepressants can increase these symptoms in children, teens, and young adults. Cymbalta is not approved for children under 18 [voiceover occurs as an older man is shown camping with his family, cooking by the fire, as the family is smiling and laughing]. People taking MAOIs or Thioridazine, or with uncontrolled glaucoma, should not take Cymbalta. Taking it with NSAID pain relievers, aspirin, or blood thinners may increase bleeding risk [voiceover occurs as an older couple is shown holding hands in their home, kissing each other playfully, then looking out a window together]. Severe liver problems, some fatal, were reported. Signs include abdominal pain and yellowing of the skin or eyes [voiceover occurs while a family is shown walking along a small crick, fishing together and having conversations while smiling]. Talk with your doctor about your medicines, including those for migraines, or if you have fever, confusion, or stiff muscles, to address a possibly life-threatening condition [voiceover occurs as a young woman is shown tranquilly reading a book outside while smiling]. Tell your doctor about alcohol use, liver disease, and before you reduce or stop taking Cymbalta. Dizziness or fainting may occur upon standing. Side effects include: nausea, dry mouth, and constipation [voiceover occurs as a father is shown giving his daughter a piggy-back ride in their home, laughing and smiling while playing with her]. Ask your doctor about Cymbalta. Depression hurts – Cymbalta can help (Eli Lilly 2010a).

This particular Cymbalta advertisement aired 43 times during the data collection period, showing the reach and repetitiveness of the brand's initiative. Rather than emphasizing the use of negative emotions for this advertisement – for example showing images of the negative aspects of depression (sadness, loneliness, helplessness) – this ad conveys the "after" associated with obtaining the prescription, leading consumers to believe that not only can depression symptoms be alleviated by taking this medicine, but that personal relationships can and will improve as well.

Advertisements were also coded for other uses of emotion. The use of humor in pharmaceutical advertisements for this study also decreased significantly from the original findings of Frosch et al. (2007), with only 5.6% of advertisements conveying this emotional appeal. Conversely, the use of fantasy (operationalized as a depiction of an unrealistic or surreal scene) increased from 22.5% to 30.6%, while sex (8.3%) and nostalgia (8.3%) increased as well, perhaps showing how the pharmaceutical industry is, again, utilizing story development, emotion, and attempts at evoking particular feelings from consumers in order to sell more prescriptions. It is important to note that no controls were put in place for ad frequency, meaning that, for example, Viagra may have been advertised more during a particular time period.

Lifestyle Portrayals

Frosch et al.'s (2007) study relied on inductive coding to develop themes related to lifestyle portrayals in the advertisements collected for their sample. Inductive coding refers to the contextualization of raw, textual data into a summarized format while establishing clear links between the evaluation and/or research objectives and the summary findings derived (Bryman and Burgess 1994; Dey 1993; Thomas 2006). This technique allows a framework to be developed for the themes apparent in raw data sets (Erlandson et al. 1993; Thomas 2006). The five themes related to lifestyle portrayals in Frosch et al.'s research included: (1) does the condition interfere with desired lifestyles; (2) does the drug enable desired lifestyles; (3) is lifestyle change an option for mitigating the condition; (4) is lifestyle change framed or discussed as insufficient; and (5) is lifestyle change offered as a supplement strategy with the drug's use. They found that 30.3% of advertisements framed a condition as interfering with healthy or recreational activities for individuals. Medication was portrayed as having the ability to enable healthy or recreational activities in 56.2% of the sample. In their sample, no ads suggested that a lifestyle change could be an alternative to consuming the medication, and, in fact, 21.3% of ads claimed that lifestyle change would be insufficient. Claims that lifestyle change would be adjunct to the product's use were found in 22.5% of ads.

For this book, the same five themes developed by Frosch et al. were tested in order to update DTCA literature, with two additional informational categories included (animation and financing offers). Table 3.5 shows these same five themes in the updated sample. Two-thirds (66.7%) of the advertisements portrayed the medical condition as interfering with healthy or recreational activities, a more than doubling of Frosch et al.'s 30.3% finding. The majority (91.7%) of advertisements portrayed characters as being enabled to participate in more healthy or recreational activities as a result of having the medication, emphasizing the personal benefits associated with consumption, again a very large increase from 56.2% in Frosch et al.'s sample. This points to a discrepancy between DTCA educating the public on a health condition versus its ability to emphasize strategic advertising tactics in order to make a product more appealing, highlighting another aspect of pharmaceutical fetishism. For example, two ad versions for Lyrica, prescribed for Fibromyalgia and nerve pain, show the ability to participate in more healthy or recreational activities upon consuming the medication. Version one featured an older woman discussing her ongoing pain and fibromyalgia as she is sitting in a seamstress shop, holding her limbs in pain as she is trying to design a dress. As the side effects for Lyrica are discussed, the woman is shown back at work, extremely active, happy, and excited while designing a new, brighter dress. She addresses the camera directly and says "I learned that Lyrica can provide significant relief for fibromyalgia pain, so now, I can do more of what I love" (Pfizer, 2010a). Version two for Lyrica shows an older woman describing "My muscles ached all over. I felt this deep, lingering pain that was a complete mystery to me. My doctor diagnosed it as Fibromyalgia" (Pfizer, 2010b). The following scenes show her working in a bakery, having great difficulty while trying to ice a cake. The woman is visibly upset and frustrated. After the voiceover describes Fibromyalgia, a new scene features the woman laughing, happy, and productive in the bakery, much more active and joyful. The advertisement ends with the woman looking directly at the camera and saying "With less pain, I can do more during my day…how sweet is that?" (Pfizer 2010b).

Consistent with Frosch et al.'s (2007) findings, none of the advertisements offered lifestyle change as an alternative to product use, while 5.6% addressed lifestyle change as insufficient, and 19.4% suggested that lifestyle change adjunct to product use would be appropriate. Although these are a decrease from the earlier sample, it is unclear if the diversity of lifestyle changes has changed. In the current sample, such changes were limited in scope and arguably uncontroversial. In the cases where lifestyle change is mentioned, it is always referred to as maintaining a healthy diet with an exercise regimen.

MEDICATION PORTRAYALS

Frosch et al.'s (2007) study relied on inductive coding to develop seven themes related to medication portrayals in DTC advertisements: loss of control; regaining control; social approval; distress; product is a breakthrough in medical science; increased endurance as a result of taking a medication; and the ability for a product to prevent some type of health risk for an individual.

Instances of losing or gaining control were specifically categorized according to what was the catalyst for that control – the health condition (educational component of the advertisement) or the prescription drug (the product being sold). In Frosch et al.'s study, 67.4% of advertisements portrayed characters losing control of their own life, a loss caused by their health condition. Regaining control as a result of product use occurred in 88.8% of ads. Social approval upon consuming a medication was also high, being portrayed in 83.1% of the ads. Characters were shown being distressed as a result of their condition in 53.9% of the ads. The prescription drug was presented as being a medical breakthrough 67.4% of the time. Characters were featured as having increased endurance in 12.4% of ads as a result of taking a medication, and 11.2% featured the medication as a form of protection from a particular health risk.

Table 3.5 shows these themes in the current sample. In 52.8% of advertisements, characters were portrayed as losing control in association with having a particular health condition. This is a decrease from Frosch et al.'s finding of 67.4%, which may again be indicating the pharmaceutical industry's increase in positive emotional appeals associated with these advertisements. This claim is supported by the finding that nearly all ads in this dataset (97.2%) featured a character that regained control as a result of product use, which is an increase from the 88.8% featuring this from Frosch et al.'s study. Rather than emphasizing the negative effects associated with one's medical condition, pharmaceutical advertising focuses more on the benefits associated with product use. Thus, as the pharmaceutical industry continues to claim that its advertising serves as a form of education for consumers regarding particular health ailments, this study shows that, in terms of the ability to have control in one's own life, most often the industry emphasizes the product or the brand more so than the health condition. This finding emphasizes that an additional benefit can be gained by obtaining a prescription – not just better health, but perhaps, an increased sense of empowerment and agency in one's life. Additionally, social approval in these advertisements decreased since the original study, from 83.1% to 58.3%, once again emphasizing the focus on the individual in these advertisements. While characters are often shown enjoying their lives more, and portrayed as experiencing significantly more happy and fulfilling relationships, social approval or encouragement are not aspects of these advertisements. Instead, characters are shown as autonomous, strong, independent, and self-sufficient – having ultimate control over their health care. Interestingly, the use of "before" situations depicting the distress associated with a condition increased in this sample (66.7%), while the claim that a medication is a breakthrough decreased (41.7%).

A notable finding in the portrayals of these medications relates to perceived endurance and protection from other health risks. While only 12.4% of Frosch et al.'s (2007) sample featured characters that had increased endurance as a result of taking a medication, this study found that 72.2% of advertisements featured an increase in endurance and individual ability, signifying the autonomous, personalized, and individualized nature of these advertisements. Boniva, prescribed for Osteoporosis, features actress Sally Field becoming more active and vibrant after the brand name is introduced, as she is playing with a dog on the dock of a lake, running, and laughing. Additionally, Boniva's advertisement claims that not only can it stop bone loss, but that it can reverse it as well (Roche Group 2010). Medications portrayed as having the ability to prevent an individual from having a health ailment or disease increased substantially in this sample (72.2%) versus the findings of Frosch et al. (11.2%). For example, Plavix featured two advertisement versions in this sample, each emphasizing that a heart attack "may be lurking," emphasizing how the prescription medication offers "greater protection" and "helps to save lives" (Bristol-Myers Squibb Co. 2010a; Bristol-Myers Squibb Co. 2010b). This finding signifies the pharmaceutical industry's ability to suggestively sell medications to individuals when they may not have an immediate need for it, yet by the use of fear appeals, are sought to believe they could still benefit from asking their doctor about the prescription.

The goal of this chapter was to extend previous research on DTCA as a problematic educational venue, especially the framing of information versus the use of emotional appeals, ultimately finding that the most popular of these promotional forms reinforce social trends of commercialized health care through normalized representations of the benefits of consumption.

The results of this study show how the problematic characteristics noted by Frosch et al. (2007) have for the most part continued – or in many cases increased – in this more recent sample, solidifying even further that pharmaceutical advertisements rely far more on emotional appeals than educational appeals in their attempts to sell medicine to consumers.

To summarize, this study found that the overall length of individual DTC advertisements has increased since Frosch et al.'s original study, although this may be an artifact of different approaches to data collection. Pharmaceutical advertisements have continued to feature characters before and after they consume a medication, with an increase in the use of positive emotions and lifestyle portrayals shown after a character consumes a medication, signifying an increase in the industry's ability to positively associate their brand with a happier, healthier life. The majority of pharmaceutical advertisements in this study featured the narration of a medical disclaimer and/or presentation of side effects as a character was being shown only after consuming a prescription drug, portraying their positive experiences with drugs while the advertisements themselves are attempting to warn consumers of potentially harmful effects. DTC advertisements have increased presentations of the biological nature of mechanism of particular diseases or illnesses; however, this study operationalized this differently than Frosch et al. originally did, including any mention of the negative attributes associated with a health ailment as being informative. In cases where specific populations at a higher risk of developing certain diseases and/or ailments were addressed, the terms used in DTC advertisements were extremely vague, for example, referring to "men" or "women."

Positive emotional appeals are continuing to be used in DTC advertisements since Frosch et al.'s original study, yet negative emotional appeals in the current dataset decreased considerably, highlighting how the pharmaceutical industry has attempted to have consumers identify most with the positive, beneficial aspects of particular drugs. While the use of humor decreased in advertisements, emotional portrayals of fantasy, sex, and nostalgia minimally increased since the original study of Frosch et al. Advertisements featuring a medical condition as interfering with healthy or recreational activities more than doubled in the current study, with the majority of advertisements featuring characters enabled to participate in life events as a result of consuming a medication. Medication was portrayed as having the ability to help one regain control over their life, which featured an increase since Frosch et al.'s study. Rather than emphasizing the negative effects associated with one's medical condition, pharmaceutical advertising focused more on the benefits associated with product use.

Thus, as the pharmaceutical industry continues to claim that its advertising serves as a form of education for consumers regarding particular health ailments, this study shows that, in terms of the ability to have control in one's own life, the industry often emphasizes the product or the brand more so than the health condition. This instance becomes even greater when considering monopolies present in the pharmaceutical industry. AstraZeneca, Bayer, Merck, and Pfizer are all quick to flash their corporate logos on the screen, arguably providing a prescription drug with more clout due to brand recognition. One of the most notable findings featured in this study is the large increase seen in the portrayals of increased endurance resulting from consuming a prescription drug, signifying the individualized nature of pharmaceutical advertising. Finally, this study found an increase in the ways that DTCA frames a prescription drug as having the ability to serve as a form of prevention from a potential disease or health complication, emphasizing the use of fear appeals in instances that may not require immediate action or need.

This empirical research is useful in that it provides an empirical foundation from which important discussions can be had regarding the content of pharmaceutical advertisements and the conceptions of health being sold to consumers. However, DTC advertisements raise other, more critical questions surrounding how these advertisements construct meaning about health care treatment options, the role that prescription drugs play in health care, and even the nature of such issues as human well-being and the role of gender and age in society. While this analysis has provided a broad range of quantifiable data, perhaps the whole story is not being told, as these advertisements can serve as examples of how the prescription drug industry influences the ways in which patients develop their understandings of health, disease, and treatment.

The following chapter will look more holistically at the type of lifestyle being sold along with prescription drugs in these advertisements. It will argue that it is not one factor that makes these messages problematic, but rather a series of reoccurring images and portrayals (i.e. age, animation, branding, gender, etc.) that have permitted health care to not only become commercialized, but for this commercialization to become normalized within Western society. This means that pharmaceutical advertisements are not only signifying a product for sale to audiences, but they are also signifying cultural meaning in terms of how drug-based health care should operate on individual and social levels.

Most notably, the categories of medication and lifestyle portrayal lend themselves to further critical analysis emphasizing pharmaceutical fetishism. By offering both a quantitative, empirical and a qualitative, message-oriented analysis on DTC advertisements, this frames the commercial nature of mass culture and its impact on society. Such triangulation will highlight the forms of the system of ideology that exists within health advertising culture, forms that encompass commercial versions of the beliefs, values and aspirations of an audience to ultimately persuade them into performing a behavior of purchasing (Turow and McAllister 2009).

Chapter 4

DTC Advertisements

A Triangulated Approach

The previous chapter showed, via quantitative approaches and content analysis, how many of the problematic characteristics associated with previous DTCA research have increased, finding that pharmaceutical advertisements relied more on emotional than informational appeals when trying to sell consumers prescription drugs. This was illustrated through such variables as ad length, story structure, and length of side effect information narrated; factual claims about a target condition; appeals; lifestyle portrayals; and medication portrayals. However, no single approach may completely offer an understanding of complex cultural artifacts such as DTCA. It is instructive to apply a more critical lens at the content of these advertisements in order to determine how cultural meaning is being signified. By first offering a quantitative, empirical foundation for more critical variables included in this study, a qualitative framework can then permit the results of the analysis to be contextualized and nuanced. This chapter, therefore, highlights the textual themes offered in pharmaceutical advertisements while relying on a more critical trajectory, thereby laying the groundwork for the following chapter to discuss how pharmaceutical fetishism is promoted via a consumerist lens of the pharmaceutical industry.

The goal of this chapter is to critically evaluate and understand pharmaceutical advertisements as commercial and ideological texts, in order to more fully understand the degree to which these promotional forms reinforce or perhaps question social trends of commercialized health care. The majority of DTCA research has emphasized its use of emotional appeals and increased cases of prescribing by doctors. This text is aiming to more directly interpret the meanings of the most popular ads themselves, in an effort to describe and comprehend the ways in which the pharmaceutical industry is framing conceptions of health in the United States. This chapter relies on quantitative and qualitative research, although the focus is on the cultural elements of DTC advertisements themselves. The quantitative portion of this chapter utilizes content analyses of the more critical variables added to Frosch et al.'s (2007) original sample, with subsequent qualitative, textual analyses used to deconstruct issues of representation and the construction of personhood seen in these advertisements. For the purposes of this book, it is important to identify what makes something a critical variable. I argue that a variable is critical if it consists of cultural elements that represent issues of power. When framed this way, cultural representations can be identified via textual deconstruction, as texts inherently contain multiple modalities from which meaning is inferred. In the case of DTC advertisements, the power is the celebration of the commodity, which leads to pharmaceutical fetishism. Pharmaceutical advertisements are not only signifying a product for sale to audiences, but they are also signifying cultural meaning in terms of how health care should operate and what cultural norms should be re-appropriated within society in regards to social elements such as gender, age, and relationships.

CRITICAL FOUNDATIONS

As discussed in chapter two, the majority of DTCA research has utilized quantitative approaches to advertising content, including content analysis and experimental design. In the case of content analysis, such methods are effective at summarizing content trends of manifest content. But individual audience members experience particular media texts one at a time, with the specific narrative and cultural characteristics of a singular text often triggering significant meaning in viewers. Content analysis may not fully capture the complexity of audio-visual texts that often use subtle and com-plex signification to influence meaning. More interpretive methods which emphasize the depth of symbolic complexity may raise other elements in discussing the potential implications of DTCA for our understanding for health care.

Quantitative research utilizing content analysis may still be used to track more variables more typically seen with cultural and interpretative methods. Typically, content analyses of DTC advertisements, as illustrated in the pre-vious chapter, focus on variables that assess the level of educational infor-mation present in order to assess whether pharmaceutical marketing is FDA compliant, and also in an effort to address the "education vs. persuasion" debate referred to in chapters two and three of this book. Other quantitative studies have broadened what they code for in ways that are arguably more latent and concordant with cultural approaches, allowing for the analysis of more cultural variables. Welch Cline and Young (2004) conducted a content analysis of all DTC advertisements found in 18 popular magazines from January 1998 to December 1999 (featuring 994 DTC advertisements for 83 unique drugs), coding for the use of models, identity rewards, and relational rewards. Identity rewards included whether models appeared to be healthy, active, or friendly, and relational rewards included social context (family, romantic, work, recreational, or other) and relational context (individual alone, dyad interaction, or group of more than two people).

Although the informational content of DTC advertisements is extremely important for making educated health care decisions, it may not be the most important feature when compared with identity and relational rewards associated with products, as these components can act as forms of observational learning for individuals (Welch Cline and Young 2004). The results showed that 91.8% of advertisements depicted exclusively healthy appearing individuals, 60.4% depicted identity-rewarding levels of activity (with physical activity occurring most frequently), and 72% of ads depicted at least one person smiling (Welch Cline and Young 2004). Overall, 96.7% of the advertisements depicted at least one identity reward, showing the ways in which even a print version of an advertisement can present strong visual cues for consumers.

Schooler, Basil, and Altman (1996) found that, in billboard advertisements, consumers were exposed to identity and relational motivators, both of which contribute to forms of social learning. Specifically, billboards for alcohol and cigarettes featured more forms of social modeling than any other products, with identity motivators being defined as using more attractiveness cues and relational motivators featuring social rewards as a result of product use. This means that having the ability to symbolically associate value with a medication goes beyond basic conceptions of health, whereas controlling a condition becomes synonymous with controlling one's identity (Charmaz 1991).

Since this chapter uses both quantitative and qualitative measures to more critically address issues of representation in DTC advertisements, it is important to also review qualitative research conducted on this subject, although such research is scarcer than qualitative. The need for more critical research on DTCA has been researched, as one study examined ten years' worth of articles from 11 academic journals in order to assess the nature of research on this topic (Pearce and Baran 2008). Researchers found that out of 16 articles written on DTCA, none were critical in nature, pointing to the need for this type of research. Critical research has been since published on the subject, addressing the importance of taking more critical approaches toward health care deconstruction.

Landau (2011) analyzed visual and verbal instances of presence and absence in two videos for Merck's "Tell Someone" DTC campaign, which problematically argues that women will get cancer if the human papilloma-virus (HPS) is contracted. By presenting a limited course of health preven-tion, and disguising the advertisement as a public health campaign, Landau found that DTC advertisements often serve as forms of masked education, thereby presenting patients with information that is not only inaccurate, but unclear, coming from a corporately branded lens that simultaneously permits the female body to be commodified. Barker (2011) also looked at gendered forms of DTC advertisements, conducting a narrative analysis of Lyrica's marketing campaign alongside the responses of fibromyalgia suf-ferers to the medication's advertisements. By demonstrating the symbiotic relationship between the pharmaceutical industry's interests, medicalization, and instances of contested illness, Barker found that illnesses perceived as less legitimate by the public are advertised in a way that equates women with irrationality (Barker 2011).

Qualitative research has also evaluated patient perceptions of DTC advertisements, with one study in particular (Zubow Poe 2012) examining the responses of 25 older women (ages 65–90) who were found to act as health information seekers for themselves and their families. Participants were shown 12 print versions of DTC advertisements aimed at older con-sumers and in-depth interviews were conducted. The study found that four "health media filters" were used by participants to help them understand the symbolic texts and pictures in the ads (Zubow Poe 2012), including relatable lived health experiences; observations made on behalf of health concerns for family members, friends, or associates; a reflection containing feelings about individual healthcare provider experiences and competence; and see-ing drug companies as credible and valuable sources of health information. The tendency for participants to "filter" each advertisement for immediate personal relevance could align with the meaning-making abilities of these advertisements for health care consumers. Qualitative research has also examined physician perceptions of DTCA. In one study based on in-depth interviews and critical discourse analysis, authors found that physician con-cerns regarding DTCA persist, with the most frequent concerns including patients acquiring a false sense of autonomy and making more requests for unnecessary or more expensive drugs (Germeni et al. 2013).

The previous research cited suggests that DTC advertisements attract the attention of consumers focusing on messages that invite a particular identifi-cation with depictions, associate rewards with these depictions, and suggest that a reward can be gained by obtaining a particular advertised drug (Welch Cline and Young 2004). Being that research has shown the potential for observational learning that DTCA features, it is all the more important to look critically at the content of these advertisements in an effort to further understand exactly what types of messages are being promoted to consumers.

Infusing emotional situations with rhetorical appeals designed to heighten the emotional impact of an advertisement (and its subsequent interpretation by the consumer) is certainly problematic if not outright deceptive, suggesting a dubious relationship between advertising's ostensible and actual intent. There is also the potential for patients to see these advertisements as a "quick-fix" for health ailments, leading them to believe that one pill can provide a remedy without encouraging serious consideration of potential side effects or risks. One study found that the benefits of a drug were delivered to suit a lower grade level of literacy (sixth grade), whereas the side effects presented are more suited for a higher grade level of literacy (ninth grade) in order to be comprehended by consumers (Kaphingst et al. 2004). Such findings suggest that, rather than educating consumers on drugs and their potential side effects and risks, advertisers prioritize revenue over social responsibility, an especially serious concern given that prescription drugs can cause serious health hazards, and in the most serious of cases, death.

In order to best address how to critically analyze DTC advertisements, this chapter is informed by grounded theory, which looks at how texts are produced, what meanings are embedded, and examines the structure, in an effort to discover common thematic categories that aide in asking the appropriate questions for analysis (Glaser and Straus 1967). Grounded theory is a qualitative, systematic, and flexible method that approaches the collection and analysis of data to construct theories "grounded" in the data themselves (Charmaz 2006). Coding of the most common themes seen in the dataset helped to shape an analytic framework for further analysis. In grounded theory, coding is the first step in attempting to define what is happening in the data, followed by the development of an emergent theory to explain the data (Charmaz 2006; Glaser 1978; Glaser and Strauss 1967). Grounded theories that utilize textual analysis can address the form of a text as well as its content, audiences, and production or presentation aspects (Charmaz 2006).

Textual analysis is often used alongside grounded theory and involves the deconstruction of the discourse in and surrounding the artifact (in this case, DTC advertisements), thereby determining what conventions are followed and how the texts themselves with embedded signifying elements may influence meanings for audience members. Textual analyses for this study relied on the theoretical underpinnings of Consumer Culture Theory, which involves the reading of popular culture texts as forms of lifestyle and identity construction which "convey unadulterated marketplace ideologies (e.g. 'look like this, act like this, want these things, aspire to this kind of lifestyle') and idealized consumer types" (Arnould and Thompson 2005, 868). Textual analysis "can offer creative ways to articulate experiences that would otherwise be inaccessible to empirical research methods" (Phillipov 2013, 209). Furthermore, this method can be useful for discovering alternative dimensions of research that may otherwise be inaccessible when using only empirical methods (Bennett 2005; Phillipov 2013). There are many advantages to textual analysis, especially its richness in terms of close reading of texts which allows significant details to be revealed (Silverman 2006). Texts are useful for analysis because they are vehicles for human meaning, consisting of interpretations of everyday life for individuals and society (Bernard 2006). Mass produced texts, such as DTC advertisements, disseminate particular versions of reality that reinforce power (or powerlessness) of particular classes while simultaneously positioning the "other," with the other being defined by representations such as gender, sexuality, ethnicity, able-bodiedness, etc. Much of textual analysis involves placing the text within the intended context, looking at how contextual meanings the text implies, and which realities the text claims to represent (Bogard 2001). In non-health contexts, there is also a long traditional of applying textual analysis to advertising and other commercial forms (Dickinson 2005; Fiske and Hartley 1978; Goffman 1979; Stein 2002; Williamson 1978).

In order to provide an empirical foundation via descriptive statistics from which to make more critical observations, this chapter uses content analysis. As discussed in the previous chapter, researchers have described two types of content: manifest and latent. The majority of content analysis research focuses on manifest content, meaning those elements which are physically present and countable (Gray and Densten 1998). Manifest content looks at the surface of a message, whereas latent content looks at the deeper structure by inferring from symbols used. Latent content includes that which may not be measured directly, but can be represented or measured by one or more indicators (Hair et al. 1998). Original conceptions of content analysis, such as that of Berelson's (1952) description, emphasize the use of manifest content only, but research now promotes the use of latent constructs as a way of integrating quantitative and qualitative analyses (Gray and Densten 1998). Content analysis is used to describe the manifest content of the dataset, while the latent content is analyzed via grounded theory and textual analysis. The findings of this study are provided via textual analyses and the following chapter will offer greater context of a particular drug featured in this dataset that decodes one advertisement using critical theory. As this portion of the research is utilizing the same dataset from the previous chapter, the same sampling strategies were utilized. As noted earlier, the dataset for this discussion comes from a convenience sample of 36 unique broadcast television DTC advertisements from 2010 collected for a separate study (see Table 4.2 for prescription drug advertisements captured).

Grounded theory was used to develop common thematic categories for these questions. Open and axial coding were used in order to define common

Table 4.1 Quantitative Proportion of Advertisements that Present Critical Variables Defined via Grounded Theory

Categories of Content in Advertisements	Percentage of Category Representation Out of 36 Unique Advertisement Versions	Number of Airings of Ads Containing Representation Category out of Total n Airing of 1,656
Gender Roles		
Characters portray "traditional" gender roles	30.6	257
Character Age		
Older adult perceived as more active as a result of taking medication	58.3	474
Appeals		
Nuclear family activities	38.9	259
Character Relationship		
Romantic heterosexual relationship portrayed	36.1	318
Physician Portrayal		
Physician portrayed	19.4	132
Actor used as physician	11.1	107
Actual physician testimonial	5.6	9
Doctor-patient interaction portrayed	16.7	126
Patient Portrayal		
Patient/user of medication portrayed	94.4	786
Patient/user of medication speaks directly to camera	63.9	516
Actor used as patient	80.6	722
Actual patient used	11.1	64

*Note: n for each category varies in accordance with the percentage out of all ads aired, as each prescription drug advertisement included in this dataset aired with varied frequency. See Table 4.2 for the number of times each ad version aired.
Source: Table created by Janelle Applequist.

themes, which were then quantitatively analyzed. Main characters were identified for each advertisement based on the length of time featured in the commercial and their narrative role. Based on the method of grounded theory, upon analyzing the dataset for thematic content, categories for analysis were created. Thematic concepts that emerged were discussed among the lead author and two volunteer coders, which led to the creation of specific coding categories. For this study, the following categories were generated based on the thematic analysis in order to extend previous research: (1) gender – traditional gender roles are portrayed in the advertisement, that is, a woman is

Table 4.2 Number of Times Each Advertisement Aired during Capture Period, with Total Advertisement Airings (*n*) = 1,656

Prescription Brand Name and Ad Version	Manufacturer	Advertised Indication	Number of Times Ad Aired during Sample Period (Total n for All Ads = 1,656)
Abilify (version 1)	Bristol-Myers Squibb Co.	Depression	6
Abilify (version 2)	Bristol-Myers Squibb Co.	Depression	8
Advair (version 1)	GlaxoSmithKline	Asthma, COPD	61
Advair (version 2)	GlaxoSmithKline	Asthma, COPD	14
Advair (version 3)	GlaxoSmithKline	Asthma, COPD	3
Avodart	GlaxoSmithKline	BPH (Benign Prostatic Hyperplasia)	25
Boniva	Roche Group	Osteoporosis	14
Avodart	GlaxoSmithKline	BPH (Benign Prostatic Hyperplasia)	25
Cialis (version 1)	Eli Lilly	Erectile Dysfunction	51
Cialis (version 2)	Eli Lilly	Erectile Dysfunction	1
Crestor (version 1)	AstraZeneca	High cholesterol, Atherosclerosis	55
Crestor (version 2)	AstraZeneca	High cholesterol, Atherosclerosis	4
Cymbalta	Eli Lilly	Depression	43
Lipitor (version 1)	Pfizer	High cholesterol, high triglycerides, stroke & heart attack prevention	39
Lipitor (version 2)	Pfizer	High cholesterol, high triglycerides, stroke & heart attack prevention	5
Lovaza	GlaxoSmithKline	High triglycerides	14
Lunesta	Dainippon Sumitomo Pharma. Ltd.	Insomnia	8
Lyrica (version 1)	Pfizer v	Fibromyalgia	38

Lyrica (version 2)	Pfizer	Fibromyalgia	1
Nasonex	Merck	Seasonal & perennial allergies	65
Omnaris	Dainippon Sumitomo Pharma. Co. Ltd.	Seasonal & perennial allergies, Allergic Rhinitis	47
Plavix (version 1)	Bristol-Myers Squibb Co.	Stroke & heart attack prevention	42
Plavix (version 2)	Bristol-Myers Squibb Co.	Stroke & heart attack prevention	42
Restasis (version 1)	Allergan Inc.	Chronic dry eye	6
Restasis (version 2)	Allergan Inc.	Chronic dry eye	3
Seroquel XR	AstraZeneca	Bipolar Depression, Schizophrenia, Depression	12
Simponi	Janseen Pharmaceuticals	Rheumatoid Arthritis, Psoriatic Arthritis	14
Spiriva	Boehringer Ingelheim Inc.	Emphysema, Chronic bronchitis, COPD (Chronic Obstructive Pulmonary Disease)	7
Symbicort (version 1)	AstraZeneca	Asthma, Chronic bronchitis, COPD (Chronic Obstructive Pulmonary Disease)	33
Symbicort (version 2)	AstraZeneca	Asthma, Chronic bronchitis, COPD (Chronic Obstructive Pulmonary Disease)	23
Symbicort (version 3)	AstraZeneca	Asthma, Chronic bronchitis, COPD (Chronic Obstructive Pulmonary Disease)	8
Toviaz	Pfizer	Overactive bladder	31
Trilipix	Abbott Laboratories	High cholesterol, high triglycerides	27
Vesicare	Astellas Pharma. Inc.	Overactive bladder	16
Viagra	Pfizer	Erectile dysfunction	9
YAZ	Bayer	Birth control, Premenstrual Dysphoric Disorder (PMDD)	23

Note: Table created by Janelle Applequist.

cooking or a woman is working on car repairs; (2) age of characters – is an older adult presented as more active as a result of taking the medication?; (3) family structure – how are families organized and portrayed in the context of DTCA?; (4) relationship portrayal – intimate relationship present is heterosexual; (5) patient portrayals – testimonial versus paid actor; and (6) physician portrayals – testimonial versus paid actor. The author, one master's level research assistant, and one bachelor's level research assistant were trained for two hours each and coded all of the advertisements independently. The quantitative results provided an empirical foundation from which to perform textual analyses highlighting more critical orientations.

Textual analyses complemented the quantitative coding process used for this chapter in that it aides in the ability to describe the nuances present in DTC advertisements, primarily shown via categories of representation and patient portrayals. By deconstructing these texts, the ways in which capitalist cultural production systems invade identity and lifestyle formation of consumers can be shown (Arnould and Thompson 2005).

This chapter addresses what types of characters are portrayed in pharmaceutical advertisements and what subsequent issues of power can be viewed as a result. This inquiry is useful in that it can shed light on the ways in which the pharmaceutical industry not only views consumers (or at least how the industry wants the consumers to view themselves), but in what ways niche markets are being targeted using specific representations and appeals. Therefore, this chapter attempts to answer what types of patients are featured in pharmaceutical advertisements. Second, issues of power are examined as seen through the process of "othering" in pharmaceutical advertising, namely via issues of representation, as discussed earlier in this chapter.

For the quantitative content analysis portion of this chapter, good aggregate intercoder reliability was found for coding categories, as indicated by K (Cohen's kappa) values ranging from 0.88–0.91 (Cohen 1960; Cohen 1968; Neurendorf 2002). For all cases ($n = 1,656$) and decisions ($n = 4,968$), the average pairwise agreement among the three coders was 95.0%, with the overall average K value being 0.89. Cohen's kappa accounts for chance agreement with the added benefit of accounting for differences in the distribution of values across categories for different coders (Cohen 1960; Cohen 1968). Specific coding categories were developed for this study using grounded theory and thematic analysis, with respective results via content analysis shown in Table 4.1 and textual analyses interpretations discussed below.

As this chapter framed DTC advertisements through a more critical lens, it is important to consider multiple issues of representation that were seen as emergent thematic categories, including issues related to gender, age, familial depictions, sexual relationships, and labels of "physician" and/or "patient."

GENDER ROLES

This chapter operationalized gender roles as the performance of particular stereotypes that exist, creating certain expectations for male and female behavior. "Traditional" gender roles were conceptualized as those that framed males as more aggressive, independent, task-oriented, and masculine, whereas females were portrayed as more sensitive, emotional, gentle, dependent, people-oriented, and service-oriented (Burn 1996). Typically, service-oriented approaches to gender stereotypes feature females as responsible for the cleanliness and maintenance of the domestic sphere, including the responsibilities of cleaning their home, cooking, and raising children, and this study conceptualized gender roles as being portrayed through these instances as well (Burn 1996). It is important to note that in all portrayals of a character performing a specific activity, every instance featured a character performing a more traditional form of gender via more masculine or feminine socialized roles. These specific gendered activities were shown in 30.6% of advertisements, showing the pharmaceutical industry's reliance on normalized assumptions regarding identity in order to make consumers more likely to personally associate or identify with a brand. Gendered representations were overwhelmingly present for women, pointing to the abilities of television and advertising in constructing gender identity (refer to earlier cites about gender in chapter two) (Mankekar 1993). In particular, this dataset featured multiple representations of women in traditional, domestic roles; however, these roles were positioned in a way that featured the characters as having increased agency, thereby creating a "domestic goddess" in association with the prescription drug brand (Hollows 2003). Furthermore, these advertisements align with an emphasis on character type and issues of power, in assuming a straightforward choice for women between feminism (portrayed via going after ones individual goals, being in a career setting, etc.) and domestic femininity (portrayed via cooking, sewing, childcare, etc.), whereas the gendered portrayals of males in these advertisements often show them in dual settings: in their career and referring to their family, or with their family and referring to their career.

Portrayals of women's domestic femininity became more prominent after a character obtained a drug, denoting that pharmaceuticals allow women to perform or fulfill these roles better (an enduring theme about women in consumer advertising; see Neuhaus 2011). For example, the advertisement for Simponi (a self-injectable prescription used for rheumatoid arthritis pain, stiffness, and swelling) portrayed women as being defined via another, according to the traditional gendered relationship being portrayed in the ad. First, a mother is shown taking her child to a carousel on the beach, smiling as she watches her daughter run toward the amusement park ride (Janssen

Pharmaceuticals 2010). A second sequence features a woman with her male partner on the beach, walking on the sand, and ultimately wrapping up in a blanket together, as she gazes up at him and smiles. Finally, a woman is shown shoe shopping with her female friend, laughing as she tries on a pair of red shoes, then switching to her sitting at lunch outside with her friend having a conversation. Through each of these instances, the female character is featured as having the ability to better fulfill her role as an agent dependent on another's acknowledgment – via gendered representations of women as mothers, romantic partners/wives, and shopping companions.

Alternatively, ads featured men as being able to perform domestic roles (i.e. father and spouse) while simultaneously framing these men as capable of also having a career, denoting a separate sense of agency apart from defining oneself through another's dependence. Spigel (2005) has written on how advertisements for home technologies have also used these gendered portrayals. As "posthuman domesticity" (a term used by Spigel to signify the increase in computerized and technological architectural and product designs seen in homes) is increasing, gendered patterns of labor and leisure are not only reconfigured, but also reinforced. Advertising offers a promotional rhetoric that offers freedom from their everyday reality for women trying to juggle motherhood, careers, relationships, and their homes, whereas men are targeted with portrayals that provide them with outlets to improve their own image and masculinity, ultimately framing men as having increased abilities to use technology, pursue careers, and "have it all" (Spigel 2005). Instead, advertisements serve as ways of merely redirecting types of work, not reducing them, as advertising creates additional false solutions for individuals.

Representations of women in these ads further signify how feminism is intersectional by class (Hollows 2003). In each advertisement in this dataset featuring a gendered portrayal of a woman, it is assumed that she is in a position of higher class and wealth. For example, both versions of the advertisements for Lyrica feature women in their career settings, albeit gendered career settings (a seamstress shop and a bakery), as each woman is in a position of authority and power, speaking to employees and giving them direction (Pfizer 2010a; Pfizer 2010b). This assumes that these women are of a higher class, as their positions exude a greater amount of power over those around them. In instances where more feminine depictions are used, such as that for the Cialis ad with a woman standing at the kitchen sink while washing strawberries, class is still an apparent issue, as the home used for the advertisement is lavish, perfectly organized, and obviously more expensive than what the average American could afford. Additionally, at first glance, it may seem as if the two advertisements for Lyrica place women in roles that emphasize successful business endeavors, but upon further inspection, it can be seen that portrayals of these characters as being in positions of power are what permit them to define their problems as medical in nature, thereby suggesting that all women have common symptoms that are insufficiently worthy of resolution (Barker 2011). By framing women's distress as ubiquitous under the guise of career success, Lyrica's advertisements continue the trend of defining women's health in narrow medical terms, ultimately disregarding the ways in which gender inequality negatively impacts women's health and women's health promotion efforts (Barker 2011). By simultaneously medicalizing and trivializing women's suffering, a validation of an individual's illness experience is minimized while the cultural credibility of Lyrica increases (Barker 2011).

CHARACTER AGE: OLDER ADULTS

Cognitive age involves one's self-concept, attitudes, and behaviors, with older adults who view themselves as younger being particularly attractive to advertisers, as those who "feel younger" are more likely to purchase new goods or services and are more willing to try new things (Stephens 1991). The automobile industry, recreational products, and travel services have often used the concept of cognitive age to understand their target demographics better in order to develop advertisements (Gatigon and Robertson 1985). This means that advertisers benefit from presenting older adults as younger, more active, and more affluent in order to influence the purchase of new products (Stephens 1991). This chapter confirms that pharmaceutical advertising utilizes the concept of cognitive age, as older adults are portrayed as more active and vibrant as a result of obtaining a prescription drug, aligning with this book's initial inquiry regarding what types of characters are portrayed in DTC advertisements. As these advertisements market more drugs to older adults in a way that features its actors as more active, healthy, and feeling younger, these products are simultaneously featured as ways of "fighting back" against time, further perpetuating the idea that aging in the United States is not a process where one can mature with grace and dignity (Nussbaum 2001). Research on message strategies has found that an estimated 8.5 million individuals request and receive a prescription drug from their physician in response to seeing an advertisement on television each year (Heinrich 2002), meaning that future research should look more closely at the concept of cognitive age alongside DTCA content in order to understand how advertisers are framing their consumers and the implications these advertisements may have on our society's understanding of the aging process.

This chapter shows that 58.3% of main characters (signified as described earlier via the one individual having the greatest narrative role in the ad) featured in the sample were perceived as older adults, which coders signified by the presence of graying hair, references to grandchildren, or direct references made to "getting older." This category included not only the presence of an older individual, but most interestingly, an older adult that was perceived to become more active and vibrant as a result of having a particular medication. Representations often included an emphasis on youthfulness, agility, and the ability to participate in recreational activities requiring increased endurance and strength (i.e. kayaking, playing baseball). This finding reflects important messages about growing older and the construction of DTC drugs as a "fountain of youth," ultimately finding that older adults are positioned as powerful beings with their representations signifying that growing older is something that needs to be performed successfully.

An ad for Trilipix, prescribed to treat high cholesterol, features an older woman encouraging the audience the "get the picture" if they are already taking a statin to reduce their blood pressure. She is featured through the camera lens, with each shot only featuring a close-up of her wrinkles and graying hair. As the advertisement continues, the narrator encourages that patients can "get the whole picture" by talking with their doctor about Trilipix and how it can improve all three cholesterol numbers (LDL, HDL, and triglycerides) when already taking a statin, yet, the on-screen text read simultaneously reads: "Trilipix has not been shown to prevent heart attacks or stroke more than a statin alone" (Abbott Laboratories 2010). The commercial continues by showing the main character becoming more active, vibrant, and energetic as a result of her experience with the medication. The "after" shots feature her teaching a group of students in an outside setting, as she is walking around, smiling, and calling on students who are asking questions. The use of youth in this advertisement signifies that one can become more youthful by association. She is seemingly more active following her use of the prescription drug, signifying her ability to identify more with the younger group of individuals she is teaching.

DTCA uses message strategies in an effort to appeal to younger self-images of older adults, deemed as "new age consumers," involving the development of products that meet unique needs while essentially masking age, transfiguring the courses of life into market segments that can result in higher sales. In this sense, the focus is on how old an individual feels rather than how old they actually are. While this can be positively viewed as a form of going against traditional ageist representations of older adults, it also can be viewed as confining in terms of its portrayal of growing older. Rather than emphasizing an idealized version of the elderly, pharmaceutical advertisements should investigate how images of aging can be shown without denying the real health and life quality changes one faces during their lifespan (Nussbaum 2001).

NUCLEAR FAMILY ACTIVITIES

The depiction of nuclear families consisting of a mother and father are not new conceptions for advertising culture. Historically, advertising as an industry has featured representations of commodities as having indirect resolutions to familial problems since addressing the working-class after World War II (Lipsitz 2003). In effect, advertising served as a form of mediation for conflicts between consumerist desires and family roles, similar to the ways in which advertising operates today as a source of remedying personal areas in the lives of consumers (Lipsitz 2003). Beyond having the ability to frame commodities as sources of mediation for problems, it can be argued that advertising is also effective in its ability to suggest that products can help to maintain already-existing relationships, most notably, within a family setting. Since the late 1800s, women in advertisements have predominantly been portrayed as mothers and housewives, solidifying gender roles that position "housewives" as females that complete household tasks within their busy lives as a sign of motherly love (Neuhaus 2011). As we rarely have the opportunity to witness family activities, household happenings, or parenting styles outside of our own homes, advertising offers one of the most salient examples of family for individuals in society, further signifying the importance it plays in the construction of normalized assumptions regarding the family unit.

It is clear that DTC advertisements position the family unit in a very normative ways. Previous research has argued that pharmaceutical advertisements normalize specific lifestyle-related activities, which have previously been reported to include traditional representations of sex/gender, body image, and domestic settings; showing how self-identification of one's role in their respective family unit (i.e. viewing the self as a sister, daughter, or granddaughter in addition to identifying as an individual) is a recurring theme in these advertisements (Fox and Ward 2009). With this study, nuclear family portrayals were a main component of 38.9% of the dataset, and in all cases where family interactions were shown, the family included a mother, father, children, and in some cases, grandparents. DTC advertisements feature the family as an integral component in health – that is, the ways in which one's family becomes directly or indirectly affected by an individual's disease or ailment. The incorporation of the family unit in these advertisements serves as an extension of the general pharmaceuticalization of domesticity or everyday life, showing that "cookie cutter" depictions of family are the only types featured in DTCA (e.g. nuclear, white, upper-class).

For example, in two of three versions for Advair featured in this dataset, nuclear family portrayals were the focus of the advertisement. Intended to treat COPD (Chronic Obstructive Pulmonary Disease) and asthma, each version emphasized how these conditions interfere not just with daily activities, but most importantly, with the ability to interact with family members. Version one portrays a grandmother at a family barbeque, yet only shows the "after" effects associated with using Advair (GlaxoSmithKline 2010a). She is shown running around a park with her grandchildren, picking them up and laughing, and then blowing bubbles with one of the youngest children. Each shot emphasizes her ability to not only remain active as a result of consuming the prescription, but most importantly, shows the meaningful relationships she is able to maintain while being more active, representing greater familial success, and subsequent power, is obtainable via a pharmaceutical drug in that it will make familial relationships more fulfilling. Both versions of Advair's advertisements feature grandparents with their grandchildren, driving home the point that the drug is not only necessary for fulfilling this family role, but that being a grandparent is an essential activity for the elderly. The second version features a grandfather with his grandchildren, running around a zoo, playing, being active, and excitedly pointing at animals they see together (GlaxoSmithKline 2010b). There are three shots of the grandfather chasing his grandchildren around the zoo while laughing and smiling. The first seconds of the commercial feature the grandfather exclaiming "I have COPD, which makes it hard to breathe...but now that I'm breathing better with Advair, I can enjoy the zoo with my grandkids." The advertisement features the grandfather blowing a pinwheel while with his grandchildren at the zoo, explicitly linking healthy lungs with childlike fun, as the grandchildren clap as he blows the pinwheel with his Advair-healed lungs. The commercial ends with the grandchildren exclaiming "We had a great day, grandpa" and the grandfather responding, "We sure did." This further constructs the family unit in the advertisement, equating successful aging with health, youth, and familial relationships.

CHARACTER RELATIONSHIP:
ROMANTIC HETEROSEXUALITY

Heteronormativity refers to the "placing of heterosexual experience at the center of one's attention, thereby making the routine assumption that heterosexuality is always 'normal' and any other form of sexuality can be perceived as 'deviant'" (Dines and Humez 2015, 731). Fuqua (2012) has written that stereotypical versions of males have been perpetuated via hegemonic masculinity, particularly through Pfizer's Viagra ads. Viagra, a prescription drug for erectile dysfunction (ED) simultaneously stabilizes and destabilizes male masculinity by encouraging patients to talk about their bodies and sexual lives beyond aging stereotypes, yet the advertisements also "repackage contemporary cultural ideas about hegemonic masculinity and recirculate them as discursive practices" (Fuqua 2012, 127). Previous research has looked at the ways in which Viagra's ad campaigns reinforce hegemonic masculinity by mandating that men must be heterosexual, independent, aggressive, and successful, thereby equating male sexuality with erection and physical performance, thereby maintaining gendered hierarchies of power and control (Baglia 2005; Gross and Blundo 2005; Rosenfield and Faircloth 2006). In this sense, the advertisements serve as a way of constructing intimacy as only achievable via adequate, penetrative sex, with heterosexual relationships being the only types featured, valued, and normalized, further subordinating and marginalizing other male expressions of sexuality (Baglia 2005).

Intimate relationships were featured in 36.1% of the advertisements, with every one of these instances portraying a heterosexual relationship. Coding for intimate relationships involved the portrayal of a couple: holding hands, looking affectionately at one another, lying in bed together, or kissing. As would be expected, intimate relationships were the main focus in prescription drug advertisements for erectile dysfunction (ED), such as those for Cialis; however, these portrayals were conveyed through a heteronormative lens.

Two versions for Cialis were featured in this dataset, with the first reiterating four times that "men can become more confident with Cialis" (Eli Lilly 2010b). The male partner in the advertisement is shown painting walls in his home with who is assumed to be his wife, and as the narrator begins describing the drug's dosing options, the walls of the home begin to fall down, revealing the outdoors, which features privacy in the woods, signaling a natural environment that signals intimacy and connectedness. The male is shown leading the female into the woods, which serves as a form of aggressiveness as the man is willing to "take the lead" and capture the moment. The narrator emphasizes "being ready for your moment" with Cialis, leading once again to the responsibility placed on the male to take control of their sexuality, but in a way that perpetuates hegemonic versions of what it means to be masculine. Interestingly, the female character rather than the male looks directly at the camera and narrates the side effects. This can be interpreted as using the female to soften the disclaimers, further positioning the male in a position of power and authority, as his role in terms of providing potentially lethal information is mitigated through the use of the wife. The narrative of the advertisement itself, however, is provided by a male voice, signaling the pressure put on men to perform sexually, but intimately with their partners as well. The second version of the advertisement for Cialis, again, features a male and female partner, both in the kitchen together preparing food. The female is at the sink rinsing a bowl of berries, and as the male partner touches her hand, the narrator beings discussing how "men can become more confident with Cialis" (Eli Lilly 2010c). As in the first version, the walls break down to reveal outdoor scenery, and the female partner describes the side effects for the medication directly to the camera among the more natural setting. The use of the outdoors in both ad versions for Cialis serves multiple purposes. First, the outdoor setting allows Cialis to be equated with a natural setting; signaling that the drug is natural and can become a natural component to a male's sexuality. Second, heterosexual relationships are framed as being more natural and acceptable. Finally, the use of the outdoor environment also symbolically shows how sex is getting involved with your natural, physical self, making the prescription drug seem like a more acceptable option, as it serves as a natural extension of the body.

Particularly in instances where a product claiming to increase sexual stamina are being advertised, it is important to look at the types of relationships being portrayed. Every romantic relationship featured relied on heteronormative assumptions, meaning that homosexual, bisexual, and pansexual relationships are reiterated as being outside of the "normal" scope of everyday life. As this book analyzes character portrayal and issues of representation via power, this discussion exemplifies how pharmaceutical advertisements are created for an assumed heterosexual audience, which permits a discourse to be created and perpetuated that reaffirms the most powerful audience members are heterosexual. The presence of heterosexuality, and the subsequent absence of homosexuality, bisexuality, and pansexuality, in pharmaceutical advertisements, denotes a need for viewing the commercial content within the context of the logics of control and de-politicization that have historically governed gay representation in general and extended to gay representation in the media (Dow 2001).

PATIENT AND PHYSICIAN PORTRAYALS

Not surprisingly, patients are overwhelmingly present in the advertisements (94.4%), speaking to the camera 63.9% of the time presenting the self as a peer to the viewer. Testimonials featuring actual users (explicitly labeled on screen) of the medication occurred at a percentage of 11.1%, with actual physicians offering their (always positive) opinions on a drug 5.6% of the time. In instances where actual physicians were used, text accompanied their on-screen presence to indicate that the physician had been compensated for their time. No ad featured a physician in isolation from patients, but ads did portray patients leaving their physician's office after obtaining a medication feeling visibly happier, empowered, and excited. For example, the advertisement for Viagra opens with a man talking to himself in the mirror, practicing how he will approach the sensitive subject of erectile dysfunction with his physician (Pfizer 2010d). The ad then shows the patient speaking with his doctor, immediately feeling more comfortable, and as he leaves the appointment room, he is walking down the street while smiling and looking self-accomplished. He then stops to purchase flowers, assumed to be for an intimate partner that is never shown in the ad. Conversely, 16.7% of advertisements featured scenes with a patient interacting with their physician, most often in the form of the patient speaking to their doctor, offering a look at the empowerment possible through the obtainment of a medication. The low presence of physicians being featured interacting with a patient may be indicative of the construction of health in these advertisements as only really involving two parties: the consumer/patient and the prescription drug, pointing to issues with limited character portrayal and power, as the most prominent medical authority in DTC advertisements being not physicians, but drugs and/or drug companies. In this sense, DTCA marginalizes physicians as less prominent authority figures in health care treatment, with the most prominent medical authority in the ads being the drugs and/or drug companies. A content analysis of print DTC advertisements for antidepressants from 1997–2006 found that two models of interaction between patients and physicians appear in ads: physician as confidant and consumer-and-supplier (Arney and Lewin 2013). Physician as confidant models featured a high degree of emotional connection between the physician and patient, whereas the consumer-and-supplier model impact implied a relationship based on exchange and negotiation, with both models fitting into the realm of a "shared-decision-making" model (Arney and Lewin 2013). Consistent with the results of this dataset, this model implies that the physician is not the gatekeeper of the prescription drug, but rather, that patients should become more proactive in voicing their opinions and needs with their physicians. This denotes another facet of the ways in which DTCA promotes patient individuality and autonomy as beneficial traits when attempting to make health care decisions.

The use of grounded theory in this chapter found that the theory of pharmaceutical fetishism is grounded in the dataset used, meaning that it is highly probably that the same conceptions have been used, and are continuing to be used, in DTC advertisements of pharmaceutical drugs. This chapter raises many questions regarding the content of pharmaceutical advertisements, particularly in association with issues of patient representation in advertisements. Although there were multiple findings that raise important questions for consumers, the scope of this discussion will focus on a limited number of findings in order to more descriptively address a few important issues.

Raymond Williams' influential essay, originally written in the 1960s, outlines advertising and public relations practices that are still influential today in the pharmaceutical industry. The most prominent aspect to come from Williams' work is his reference to advertising as "magic," referring to the ability of advertising to go beyond the material and appeal to the desires of individuals (Williams 1980). He critiques our culture by saying that we are, in fact, not materialist enough, as members of our society are not satisfied with the material product, but additionally need a secondary effect (e.g. clothing must only serve its functional purpose, but it also has the ability to make us feel popular, sexy, happy, etc.) (Williams 1980). Material needs are present, but individuals have other needs that go beyond the material which are far more powerful, so advertising appeals to these desires, and it must show that these desires can be fulfilled.

Pharmaceutical advertisements are explicitly utilizing the "magic" of advertising by presenting prescription drugs as cures for more than just health conditions. Drugs are advertised in a way that presents them as having the added benefit of selling a particular lifestyle to individuals – one that emphasizes happiness, successful relationships, nuclear family activities, and personal fulfillment. Furthermore, these ads perpetuate normalized conceptions of particular representations, featuring characters that portray stereotypical gender roles, youthfulness even in cases of being older, heteronormative relationships, familial relationships as being central to health, and patients as being autonomous from their physicians. This means that drugs have been commodified to sell much more than remedies for health conditions. Commodity fetishism is the relationship between people and products, and fetishism occurs once individuals see meaning in things that seem an inherent part of their physical existence, yet, the meaning is actually created by individuals themselves (Marx 1992). Thus, products appear to have value inherent in them, but the fact is that human beings themselves produce the additional value. Advertisements allow for culture to associate products with meaning, as emotional meaning, forms of promotional culture, and even logos and branding animation (i.e. the use of animation in pharmaceutical advertisements) can evoke sentiment for individuals (Williams 1980). Additionally, the production contexts for these drugs are removed from the advertisements themselves, with the product (the drug) being portrayed as heroic. By claiming that individuals are not materialistic enough, Williams is saying that advertising works because it promises to solve non-material problems. If individuals were materialistic enough, they would only look at advertisements for the informational value in order to gauge how a product can serve functional needs. Instead, individuals look for added meaning or value in products, being confronted with an advertising culture that promises to fulfill additional needs and desires. The magic, then, is that advertising tells us our desires can be met. In this sense, pharmaceutical advertisers are meeting the health needs of consumers, but also meeting their inner, more personal needs – the need to feel youthful, the need to perform, the need to be happy.

The advertisements utilize this "magic" predominantly through the use of "before and after" imagery. The most common theme seen throughout the advertisements was the lack of agency characters portrayed until they obtained the prescription drug, reiterating the message that the power to change one's life comes from the medication itself. This neo-liberal message propagates the notion that a consumable product, in this case a potentially deadly one, can make one not only a better version of themselves, but a better version than the rest of society as well. This message is exemplified through the portrayals of characters being active, youthful, participating in heterosexual relationships, and maintaining traditional gender roles.

Unfortunately, for all of the debate surrounding the diminishment of the doctor-patient relationship, problems associated with patient self-diagnosis and advertising's control over medical decisions to come as a result of pharmaceutical advertising, current policies have shifted over time to offer a false representation that these advertisements are not desecrating patients. Perhaps what is even more problematic in this sense is not necessarily the relaxed restrictions given by the FDA for DTC advertisements, but rather the content of the advertisements themselves and the ways in which they blatantly sell an ideology that privileges consumption over health to consumers. Furthermore, advertisers draw upon certain codes to produce the brands that become recognized, as creating a successful ad campaign relies on those trained in the industry to prioritize industrial interests over consumers, aligning with principles of capture theory (Bernstein 1955). The nature of DTCA is that it relies on the decentralization of the physician's role through its efforts to medicalize human problems, which encourages consumers to self-diagnose (Conrad 2007). This process shows how not just the contents of these ads encouraged increased cases of pharmaceutical fetishism, but how an ideology that emphasizes consumerism over patient understanding becomes commonplace in the field of health care.

Beyond the health risks associated with advertising prescription drugs to consumers not educated in medicine, the most serious implication to thinking of patients of consumers is the pseudo-individuality and pseudo-autonomy that emerge as a result of the health domain being defined based on market relations. Advertisements serve two functions in that they offer role models for consumers to identify with, framing constructions of individuals as they can aspire to be, while also encouraging consumers to enter the marketplace where desirable qualities and lifestyles are commodified and available for purchase (Sender 1999). Pharmaceutical advertisements are structured in a way that gives a consistent message to viewers that a prescription drug will significantly improve aspects of their lives that are not medically provable by research, yet, upon obtaining the product, it can be argued that little regarding one's lifestyle or happiness actually changes purely as a result of a medication. Thus, a false sense of agency is sold, with the triumph of pharmaceutical advertising being its ability to urge consumers to compulsively imitate the images they are viewing, where a false "freedom" to choose from products becomes a freedom to remain the same as everyone else (Horkheimer and Adorno 1972). Namely, patients are becoming ever more deeply inured in the ideology of the market regarding medical practices, as advertising shapes them for our society.

As discussed in chapter three, this book shows how the culmination of medicalization, pharmaceuticalization, and commodity fetishism can be used to explicate how the process of "pharmaceutical fetishism" is present in advertising culture. As sociological research has already established the relationships between consumerism and increased instances of medicalization and pharmaceuticalization, this book is devising the term pharmaceutical fetishism. Pharmaceutical fetishism is the process of the commodification of brand-name pharmaceutical drugs, which, via advertising and promotional culture, ignore large-scale production and for-profit motives of "big pharma" while simultaneously reiterating a brand discourse that offers individuals additionally constructed meanings and discourses which promote: medicine as a cultural authority in health care and prescription drugs as having the capability to solve individual problems beyond those for which a medicine is scientifically intended, thereby offering more benefits outside the realm of health purposes. The concept of pharmaceutical fetishism relies upon the forms of pseudo-autonomy and pseudo-individuality presented to consumers.

Commercial culture, which includes advertising, has saturated aspects of identity formation, oftentimes seamlessly, since the 1920s, as culture "asks people to think of themselves as individuals in need who require commodities to become who they are, as private competitors for plentitude in interpersonal and economic markets" (Budd, Craig, and Steinman 1999, 16). While advertising is not the sole social force that shapes identity, commercial culture continues to model individuality as supreme – Western ads are centered on making one person stand out among a group. Advertising is effective in its attempts to connect with the individuality of consumers because it recycles language, imagery, and symbols that are meaningful to those being targeted for sales (Spigel 1992, 7). The hegemonic power of commercialism, then, rests in its ability to encourage pseudo-individuality, where an individual feels they are motivated by their own personal desires, when, in fact, their motivation comes from a system of intricately designed commercial culture that encourages spending, shopping, and capitalism. (Spigel 1992).

Recall the earlier discussions of pseudo-individuality, commodity fetishism, and advertising as magic. These arguments can be applied to pharmaceutical fetishism present in DTCA, as these advertisements present consumers with romanticized portrayals regarding what benefits a prescription drug can offer and ignoring other treatment options. Rather than relying merely on the medical benefits associated with a drug designed to treat a target condition, the industry of DTCA has permitted these commercials to include "additional benefits," usually by relying on the use of emotional appeals or presentations of scenarios of those in the ads who have used the drugs. This means that the culture of prescription drugs is being reproduced, potentially suggesting to consumers that they can obtain positive attributes beyond what can be corrected in the body – for example, advertisements for antidepressants often feature all relationships as significantly improving and seeming "perfect" as a result of consuming a medication, but this is a veiled representation of a serious mental health condition and the social challenges that come along with it. In order to benefit capitalistic endeavors, the culture of pharmaceuticals has evolved into one that promises much more than it can realistically deliver for consumers. As Rose (2007) has suggested, DTCA may be an aspect of medicalization and pharmaceuticalization that creates false needs for consumers. Furthermore, false claims are presented to consumers that lead them to believe that pharmaceuticals can meet individual needs and desires. This can be described as a form of ideological appropriation, as the industry that exists to expand understandings of health is the very industry that creates false needs in a consumer-driven market (Abraham 2010).

Chapter 5

The Commercial Elements of Constructing a Drug

A Textual Analysis of a YAZ Advertisement

To provide a more in-depth look at the ways in which a prescription drug is advertised and produced, this chapter utilizes multivariate data stemming from chapters four and five, a political economy approach (methodology discussed in chapter two), critical advertising studies (addressed in chapter three), and textual analysis (methodology defined in chapter four), to deconstruct one especially noteworthy campaign, the prescription-only contraceptive YAZ.

The FDA first approved oral contraceptives in 1960, and women quickly accepted the shift in female-controlled contraceptive efforts. By the late 1960s, people referred to oral contraceptives simply as "The Pill," which to this day holds the same meanings and connotations, showing the popularity, reach, and cultural awareness of this pharmaceutical sector (Tone 2012). In the 1990s and 2000s, pharmaceutical marketing in the United States began to publicize birth control as more of an individual solution rather than a public health strategy (Siegel Watkins 2012). Historically, the messages surrounding the purposes for birth control (to prevent pregnancy) have changed, particularly since the 1990s as a result of less research and development on birth control methods (see chapter two) and the growth of "lifestyle drugs" (Siegel Watkins 2012). Lifestyle drugs are defined as those which are used for "non-health" problems that "lie at the margins of health and well-being…a wider definition would include drugs that are used for health problems that might better be treated by a change in lifestyle" (Gilbert, Walley, and New 2000, 1341). It was in the 1990s that oral contraceptives began to be advertised for uses beyond their original intent (birth control), including marketing to women that they could have shorter, lighter menstrual cycles, thereby introducing the subject of menstruation into the discussion of

"The Pill." In this sense, it can be argued that menstruation became a part of the already-medicalized process of contraception.

AN OVERVIEW OF YAZ AND DISEASE MONGERING

YAZ is an oral contraceptive (birth control pill) that was approved by the FDA in March of 2006 for the prevention of pregnancy. In October of 2006, the FDA approved YAZ for also treating Premenstrual Dysphoric Disorder (PMDD, a condition that is described as a more severe version of Premenstrual Syndrome (PMS) and is discussed below), with an approval for YAZ being used to treat acne passing in January of 2007 ("YAZ Approval History" 2014). In 2009, YAZ was the best-selling oral contraceptive on the American market, and was the 21st best-selling prescription drug (10 million prescriptions filled) that year ("Top 200 Drugs" 2010a; "Top 200 Drugs" 2010b). Sales for YAZ in 2010 exceeded $360 million (Tone 2012). In 2010, prescription contraceptive advertisement spending in the United States totaled $116 million (2.7%) out of the total $4.3 billion prescription drug ad spending (Kantar Media 2011).

YAZ is manufactured by Bayer, a German-based chemical and pharmaceutical company founded in 1863 ("Facts and figures" 2014). Perhaps best known for its invention of aspirin, Bayer applied for trademark protection ("Bayer Aspirin") in 1899 and was one of the first pharmaceutical companies to experiment with the commercialization of a drug (Jennewein, Durand, and Gerybadze 2010). In 1914, Bayer launched an advertisement campaign promoting its aspirin as a radical change in the industry of medicine. Although Bayer has longevity on the market and a rich history, the corporation has not come without its set of challenges. In 2001, Bayer was forced to pull its prescription drug Lipobay off the market after undesirably strong side effects were found in patients, damaging Bayer's reputation (Jennewein, Durand, and Gerybadze 2010). However, at about the same time, the anthrax crisis broke out, putting Bayer in the position to reclaim its notoriety. Bayer had the patent rights for Cipro, the only known antibiotic at the time able to fight the anthrax disease (Richter 2002). Rather than attempting to make a generous gesture and providing the public with the drugs necessary during a national epidemic, Bayer offered Cipro to United States authorities at the price of $1.77 per pill (half the retail price), but still a high price for 12 million Americans to pay in the event of an anthrax outbreak. Upon further negotiations, Bayer agreed to drop the price to $0.95 a pill, yet still suffered from a damaged reputation as a result of giving Americans the impression that greed was more important than public health (Richter 2002). This was not the last string of bad publicity Bayer faced, however, with the 2000s including public scrutiny over the pharmaceutical corporation's practices, ranging from their use of social media to promote high-profile prescription drugs to the public to its funding of a study in the New England Journal of Medicine whose lead author was a paid consultant for Bayer and also co-invented the patent behind the drug being described and applauded for leukemia treatment (Bernstein 2010; Jack 2011). Still, Bayer is one of the highest-profiting pharmaceutical companies in the world, with its overall sales ranking eighth in the world for 2013 in regards to sales and overall revenue (Palmer and Helfand 2014). In terms of DTCA, Bayer is one of the biggest in the business, spending $71.8 million on its media campaigns occurring in 2010 in the United States alone (Kantar Media 2011).

Bayer, the manufacturer of YAZ, spent a total $71.8 million on pharmaceutical advertisement spending in 2010, with $41.5 million of this amount spent solely on promoting YAZ for the broadcast marketplace. As will be discussed, however, YAZ – especially after the 2010 time period from which this book's sample was derived – has been a controversial drug with connections to serious side effects and the subject of numerous lawsuits against Bayer.

YAZ has been popular not just in the pharmaceutical marketplace since its introduction to consumers, but in research and the news as well. As mentioned above, YAZ became FDA approved to treat PMDD in 2006. PMDD has been cited in research as a form of "disease branding" or "disease mongering," with both terms referring to the selling of sickness, or shaping of public perception, in order to widen the boundaries of illness and grow the market for those who sell and deliver treatments (Payer 1992; Arnst 2006; Moynihan and Henry 2006; Parsons 2007; Elliott 2010a; Elliott 2010b). Arnst (2006) has written that another way of thinking of disease mongering is framing it as "the corporate-sponsored creation or exaggeration of maladies for the purpose of selling more drugs." Examples of disease branding in Western medicine are far-reaching, with medical diagnoses such as overactive bladder (previously referred to as incontinence), social anxiety disorder (known ten years ago as shyness) and erectile dysfunction (impotency) all transformed through marketing efforts to obtain a form of cultural legitimacy decreasing the necessity for convincing consumers that a drug is needed to fix any of these "conditions" (Elliott 2010b). One of the most successful examples of disease mongering involves GlaxoSmithKline's marketing of Paxil beginning in 1999. In an effort to target shy people and convince them they had a condition called social anxiety disorder, GlaxoSmithKline hired public relations firm Cohn and Wolfe to put together a "public awareness campaign" called "imagine being allergic to people," which also recruited NFL stars and celebrities in its message dissemination (Elliott 2010b). GlaxoSmithKline even hired academic psychiatrists and sent them to lecture on social anxiety disorder as a diagnosable condition in the top 25 media markets. In the two years prior to Paxil being approved by the FDA for treating social anxiety disorder, there were only approximately 50 references to the condition in the press. However, at the end of 1999, following the public relations campaign, there were over one billion references (Elliott 2010b). Today, social anxiety disorder is the third most common mental illness worldwide. Disease branding/mongering – as a concept that explains the expansion of drugs to numerous physical and psychological conditions – is clearly related to pharmaceutical fetishism – the application of drugs as a solution to numerous personal and social problems; the persuasive and communicative techniques in DTC advertisements may in fact link the two theoretical concepts in semiotic practice.

In the case of oral contraceptives being marketed to not only prevent pregnancy, but having the ability to treat PMDD, an example of corporate-sponsored exaggeration of the maladies associated with premenstrual syndrome can be seen; however, YAZ was not the first oral contraceptive to address PMDD as a treatable and diagnosable condition. In late 2000, pharmaceutical corporation Eli Lilly was faced with the prospect of losing competition to generic alternatives as its patent for Prozac was set to run out. At this time, Eli Lilly launched Sarafem, a prescription drug treatment for PMDD (Ebeling 2011). However, Sarafem and Prozac were chemically identical. Eli Lilly created a DTC marketing campaign for Sarafem in the United States that simultaneously "warned" women of the newly accepted condition known as PMDD while offering a remedy through their prescription drug. Interestingly, Eli Lilly helped to get PMDD recognized as a distinct disease, different from PMS, by the FDA in 1999 (Ebeling 2011). PMDD has been referenced as one of the most prominent examples of disease mongering in pharmaceutical advertising because of the condition's similarity to PMS, meaning that the industry took a natural bodily condition and its subsequent characteristics and exaggerated them to benefit the corporate bottom line of selling more prescription drugs (see Table 5.1 for symptoms of PMDD versus PMS). The corporation hired a clinical psychiatrist who had previously conducted clinical trials using antidepressants as a treatment for PMDD with Pfizer to provide expert testimony to the FDA's Psychopharmacological Drugs Advisory Committee (PDAC), testifying that PMDD was a disease entity and that fluoxetine (the main ingredient in Prozac) was an effective treatment for the condition (Ebeling 2011). What is arguably most concerning about the creation of PMDD as a diagnostic mental health category is the pharmaceutical industry's role in capitalizing on premenstrual experiences surrounding the marketed reinvention of PMS (Greenslit 2005). By promoting and marketing PMDD as a diagnosable condition requiring intervention, the pharmaceutical industry proved successful in defining and culturally shaping a new diagnosis, setting a precedent for this to happen again in the future.

Table 5.1   PMDD (Premenstrual Dysphoric Disorder) versus PMS (Premenstrual Syndrome)

PMDD (Premenstrual Dysphoric Disorder) Diagnostic and Statistical Manual of Mental Disorders (DSM-IV) Categorization

(A) In most menstrual cycles during the past year, five (or more) of the following symptoms were present for most of the time during the last week of the luteal phase, began to remit within a few days after the onset of the follicular phase, and were absent in the week post-menses, with at least one of the symptoms being either (1), (2), (3), or (4):

   (1) Markedly depressed mood, feelings of hopelessness, or self-deprecating thoughts
   (2) Marked anxiety, tension, feeling of being "keyed up" or "on edge"
   (3) Marked affective lability (e.g. feeling suddenly sad or tearful or increased sensitivity to rejection)
   (4) Persistent and marked anger or irritability or increased interpersonal conflicts
   (5) Decreased interest in usual activities (e.g., work, school, friends, hobbies)
   (6) Subjective sense of difficulty in concentrating
   (7) Lethargy, easy fatigability, or marked lack of energy
   (8) Marked change in appetite, overeating, or specific food cravings
   (9) Hypersomnia or insomnia (trouble sleeping)
   (10) A subjective sense of being overwhelmed or out of control
   (11) Other physical symptoms, such as breast tenderness or swelling, headaches, joint or muscle pain, a sensation of "bloating," or weight gain

(B) The disturbance markedly interferes with work or school or with usual social activities and relationships with others (e.g., avoidance of social activities, decreased productivity and efficiency at work or school).

(C) The disturbance is not merely an exacerbation of the symptoms of another disorder, such as major depressive disorder, panic disorder, dysthymic disorder, or a personality disorder (although it may be superimposed on any of these disorders).

(D) Criteria A, B, and C must be confirmed by prospective daily rating during at least two symptomatic cycles. (The diagnosis may be made provisionally prior to this confirmation.)

Source: Adapted from the American Psychiatric Association Diagnostic and statistical manual of mental disorders, 4th ed.; Bhatia and Bhatia 2002; Ebeling 2011.

*Note: For the purposes of this chapter, I italicized the common symptoms found between PMDD and PMS to show overlap and disease mongering as discussed.

PMS (Premenstrual Syndrome) Symptoms

(A) Acne
(B) *Swollen* or *tender breasts*
(C) *Feeling tired*
(D) *Trouble sleeping*
(E) Upset stomach, *bloating*, constipation, or diarrhea
(F) *Headache* or backache
(G) *Appetite changes* or food cravings
(H) *Joint* or *muscle pain*
(I) *Trouble with concentration* or memory
(J) Tension, *irritability*, mood swings, or crying spells
(K) *Anxiety* or *depression*

Source: U.S. Office on Women's Health, 2012.
Note: Table created by Janelle Applequist.

Prior to officially releasing YAZ on the market, Bayer hired global communications firm MediaEdge: Cia (MEC) to prime consumers about PMDD (Woods 2013). Upon consulting with Bayer, MEC announced that its marketing campaign had the goal of "activating girl power," creating a multimedia campaign set to "engage with young women about confidential health choices through music and online content" (Hains 2009, 98). MEC created a three-pronged, non-branded education campaign, which first consisted of hiring Australian band the Veronicas to record Twisted Sister's 1984 song "We're Not Gonna Take It," addressing the symptoms associated with menstruation. In this way, the campaign made menstrual symptoms a choice that the consumer could opt out of if they chose YAZ (Woods 2013). The second portion of the campaign involved a website, wngti.com, which was "outlined in bright pink and decorated with hearts...[and] allowed consumers to get a behind-the-scenes peek at The Veronicas and make a connection between the lyrics and their feelings about menstruation" (Woods 2013, 272). Upon visiting the site, users were given a code (understandpmdd) for a free download of the Veronicas song, and after downloading the song, were prompted to visit the third prong of MEC's campaign, which was the companion website www.understandpmdd.com. This website linked to a "body diary" (described in more details below) where women could self-diagnose PMDD and obtain a printout of their symptoms to share with their physician. Rather than presenting contraception and menstruation as natural processes associated with the female body, Bayer incorporated postfeminist depictions in its campaigns for PMDD and for its subsequent marketing of YAZ, "encouraging women to (literally) fight back against PMDD," making the obtainment of the prescription drug a means of empowerment (Woods 2013, 274). Rather than viewing menstruation and contraception efforts as issues that affect public health as a whole, Bayer encouraged women to "see menstrual suppression as a right that they can and should freely choose to exercise to gain control over their lives" (Woods 2013, 274). In addition to this campaign, Bayer also relied heavily on advertising YAZ upon its release via the medium of television broadcasting.

TEXTUAL ANALYSIS OF A TELEVISED YAZ ADVERTISEMENT

The YAZ advertisement referenced in this chapter was included in the dataset used in chapters four and five. It is important to note that prior to the airing of this advertisement in 2010, Bayer had already been sent three warning letters by the FDA claiming that three separate advertisements (from 2003, 2008, and 2009) featured false and misleading advertising claims. The letters cited that Bayer's "misleading" advertising claims were "particularly troubling" because they served to "undermine the communication of important risk information, minimizing these risks and misleadingly suggesting that YAZ is safer than has been demonstrated by substantial evidence or substantial clinical experience" (U.S. Food and Drug Administration 2008; U.S. Food and Drug Administration 2009). Table 5.2 presents the coded data for the individual YAZ advertisement in accordance with the informative/educational variables discussed in chapter four and the critical categories emphasizing representation from chapter five. For the purposes of this chapter only, both conditions most heavily advertised by Bayer for YAZ use (contraception and PMDD) were coded separately for informational/educational categories in order to differentiate which condition(s) is/are being targeted most frequently throughout the advertisement. The advertisement aired 23 times total on ABC and NBC during the time period of the sample. Thirty seconds of the advertisement's total run time of 1:10 are attributed to side effect information.

As can be seen in Table 5.2, many of the advertisement's explicit characteristics were concordant with the main results found in the previous chapter: the use of emotional appeals, positive attributes of lifestyle for those portrayed as using the drug, social approval for using the drug, an emphasis on youth, and the absence of non-pharmaceutical methods for dealing with conditions. This is true for both the contraceptive and PMDD-controlling attributes of the drug. But how do these factors manifest in the semiotic dynamics of the advertisement itself?

The advertisement opens with upbeat music playing and the viewer is able to immediately associate the commercial as mimicking a music video, as a caption appears on the bottom left-hand corner of the screen featuring the song, its artist, album name, and record label ("Change," The Veronicas, Hook Me Up, Sire Records). In this way, the commercial simultaneously attempts to deny its "commercialness" by mimicking the visuals associated with a music video, and incorporates the use of a trendy band for promotion, a common technique in modern advertising that is also increasingly embraced by the modern music industry (Taylor 2013). As this form of cross-promotion is taking place, an energetic female narrator begins to describe that "doing more, trying more, and laughing more come from your attitude, not your birth control" (Bayer 2010). As these words are spoken, the camera cuts to one-second shots of four different woman (three Caucasian and one Asian woman, all thin, all attractive, and appearing to be in their early 1920s). The first woman is shown stretching her leg at night in a park, as the camera features a close-up of her face as she looks directly at the camera, before it is presumed she will go running alone, an empowered and agentic act. The second woman is shown in her apartment, looking in the mirror while playing with her hair, contemplating whether she will change her hairstyle. She is smiling in the mirror as she lifts her hair up to see how she would like if she were

Table 5.2   Coded Data for YAZ Advertisement According to Categories Featured in Chapters Three (Informational/Educational Variables) and Four (Representation Variables)

Informational/Educational Variables	*Present in Advertisement (X Denotes Presence)*
Factual Claims (*focus on contraception)	
Biological nature or mechanism of disease	
Risk factors or cause of condition	
Prevalence of condition	
Subpopulation at risk of condition	
Appeals	
Rational	X
Positive emotional	X
Negative emotional	
Humor	X
Fantasy	
Sex	
Nostalgia	
Lifestyle Portrayals	
Condition interferes with healthy or recreational activities	X
Product enables healthy or recreational activities	X
Lifestyle change is alternative to product use	
Lifestyle change is insufficient	X
Lifestyle change is adjunct to product	
Medication Portrayals	
Loss of control caused by condition	X
Regaining control as a result of product use	X
Social approval as a result of product use	X
Distress caused by condition	
Breakthrough	X
Endurance increased as a result of product use	X

Informational/Educational Variables	*Present in Advertisement (X Denotes Presence)*
Factual Claims (*focus on PMDD)	X
Biological nature or mechanism of disease	
Risk factors or cause of condition	
Prevalence of condition	
Subpopulation at risk of condition	
Appeals	
Rational	X
Positive emotional	X
Negative emotional	
Humor	
Fantasy	
Sex	
Nostalgia	
Lifestyle Portrayals	
Condition interferes with healthy or recreational activities	X
Product enables healthy or recreational activities	X

Informational/Educational Variables	Present in Advertisement (X Denotes Presence)
Lifestyle change is alternative to product use	
Lifestyle change is insufficient	X
Lifestyle change is adjunct to product	
Medication Portrayals	
Loss of control caused by condition	X
Regaining control as a result of product use	X
Social approval as a result of product use	X
Distress caused by condition	X
Breakthrough	X
Endurance increased as a result of product use	X

Critical Variables Focusing on Representation	Present in Advertisement (X Denotes Presence)
Gender Roles	
Characters portray "traditional" gender roles	X
Appeals	
Nuclear family activities	
Character Relationship	
Romantic heterosexual relationship portrayed	
Physician Portrayal	
Physician portrayed	
Actor used as physician	
Actual physician testimonial	
Doctor-patient interaction portrayed	
Patient Portrayal	
Patient/user of medication portrayed	X
Patient/user of medication speaks directly to camera	
Actor used as patient	X
Actual patient used	

Note: Table created by Janelle Applequist.

to have bangs, as she uses her fingers to pretend she is cutting her own hair. Next, the ad features a woman laughing and smiling, as she is sitting on the edge of a bath tub filled with water and bubbles. She jokingly leans back, throwing herself into the water, fully clothed. The fourth woman is shown sitting in the back of a taxi cab, laughing at the camera as she is seated next to a variety of full shopping bags. She proceeds to smile and laugh, and leans forward closer toward the camera. The majority of the shots in this advertisement end with close-up shots of each woman, emphasizing their aesthetic beauty, flawless skin free of acne, and playful attitudes.

Each woman is shown as playful, free, and independent throughout the YAZ advertisement. The culmination of these various shots in the first six seconds of the advertisement feature emphases on independence (running alone at night), the ability to change (and seemingly improve) one's own appearance (shown in the portrayal of the hair cutting in the mirror), playfulness (leaning into a bathtub while fully clothed and being happy about doing so), and commodification (the happiness associated with purchasing products). Even in its first few seconds, it is clear that Bayer has constructed a brand, and its subsequent advertisement, that position consumers of birth control as those that are young, independent, and attractive – relying on traditional feminine representations of what it means to be a woman, simultaneously signifying who does not identify or associate with this brand as women in their 30s, 40s, or 50s (which are still demographic groups that obtain prescription forms of contraception). In this sense, YAZ equates birth control with youthfulness, insinuating that by obtaining the product, one will not only feel more playful and vibrant, but that they will give off this image to those around them as well.

The advertisement continues by featuring the logo for YAZ on screen for a three-second period (Bayer 2010). The logo simply says "YAZ," but is designed to look like it has been hand-written in a way that is carefree and not worried about perfection, which is another common theme seen throughout the portrayal of women in this advertisement. The logo itself is bright orange and easily recognizable on the screen, and for the remainder of the advertisement, it switches to the bottom left-hand corner of the screen, until the last three seconds of the commercial spot when it once again takes up the entire portion of the screen to strengthen brand association. The narrator continues speaking as the logo is shown, saying "Like all pills, YAZ is effective at preventing pregnancy and can give you shorter, lighter periods. But if you choose YAZ for birth control, it may also help treat moderate acne and Premenstrual Dysphoric Disorder, PMDD, not PMS" (Bayer 2010). Arguably, this portion of the advertisement is a form of retraction by Bayer, as they had previously been warned by the FDA about their false and misleading claims regarding the approved uses for YAZ. Rather than explicitly telling consumers this advertisement was a point of clarification for claims made in previous advertisements, though, this advertisement offers the statement as a way to "educate" consumers on the differences between PMDD and PMS. The narrator continues to speak, giving arguably important information about PMDD and its symptoms while multiple, fast-paced camera shots are continuously shown to consumers, continuing the narratives of the four characters described above. The Asian woman who was considering changing her hairstyle is shown pulling her long hair in front of her face, as she takes a pair of scissors and cuts a significant portion off in order to give herself bangs. The hair is shown falling as she cuts it off, landing on her jeans and bare feet. She then looks directly at the camera, smiling and confidently tousling her hair around with her hands, signifying her happiness with and pride in her decision to not only cut her hair, but to literally take matters into her own hands and to do it herself.

The advertisement features predominantly white women, with only one character representing a minority group (Asian). On the surface, it may seem progressive and unbiased for Bayer to use a young Asian woman as a central character in the advertisement for YAZ. Upon closer inspection, however, the use of a minority character is a form of "casting for equality," which Crockett (2008) has written is when blackness representations are used in advertisements, but done so in a way that does not make any claims about the product or viewer connecting with black cultural identity. This same argument regarding representations of African Americans in advertising can be applied to the use of an Asian character is the YAZ advertisement. In this advertisement, being Asian is represented as being devoid of any representation or examination of what it means to be a part of Asian or Asian-American culture, yet the minority presence – fully assimilated in and non-distinguishable from the majority white culture – allows the brand to associate itself with racial equality (Goldman 1992; Goldman and Papson 1996; Crockett 2008). In the ad, then, being Asian is represented as being construed via a Western reinterpretation and denotes universality to the culture of young, white women – a culture strongly associated with the use of YAZ as a key indicator of its empowered nature.

As the advertisement continues, the woman that was previously sitting in a taxi cab is shown entering the same cab (this is meant to signify a prequel to the previous depiction) and buckles her seat belt as she sets her shopping bags in the passenger seat beside her. Suddenly, as the car is moving, she begins to change her outfit, pulling a blouse over her head and placing it over her camisole. It is clear she is "getting ready on the go," (or "doing more," as the advertisement refers to repeatedly) as she removes her ponytail and shakes her hands through her hair to prepare for another event, as this shot emphasizes her appearance. Simultaneously, this depiction shows the character's ability to be confident enough to change her outfit in the back of a moving taxi cab, as she is, in a sense, taking control of the limited time she has. She proceeds to play with her hair, as she leans in closer to the camera, looking directly at the lens and giggling. Here, the advertisement implies that the woman is going from a work setting to a leisurely activity, or perhaps from an afternoon of shopping out for an evening of clubbing, as her outfit change and tousling of the hair suggests. This, then, simultaneously offers the message that the woman: (1) is headed for a night of sex, identifying with the product's ability to prevent pregnancy; (2) has great skin, as is illustrated by her movements directly toward the camera, and; (3) she in a very happy, upbeat mood, with there being no chance that her mood swings and difficulties associated with PMDD could ruin her romantic and/or social evening out. In considering the multiple modalities used in DTC advertisements, it is important to note that text is also present and constantly changing on the screen as these portrayals are being shown and the narrator is speaking.

The narrator continues to "educate" consumers on PMDD: "Unlike PMS, symptoms of PMDD are severe enough to interfere with your life" (Bayer 2010). As this is spoken, the advertisement cuts to a full-screen bulleted list titled "Emotional & Physical Symptoms of PMDD could include:" and lists items such as anxiousness, irritability, anger, headaches, bloating, and fatigue (Bayer 2010). As described earlier, these symptoms are all reported with PMS as well, pointing to a discrepancy in the advertisement's ability to clarify the differences between that and PMDD (see Table 5.1). As the list is shown on screen, a bar of text beneath reads that "YAZ is not for the treatment of PMS" and then switches to "Symptoms of PMDD occur regularly before a woman's menstrual cycle" (Bayer 2010). Once again, the advertisement fails to clarify how PMDD differs from PMS, and if pharmaceutical advertisements are meant to inform consumers of new and existing health conditions as has been previously claimed, then this topic should have been addressed in a more straightforward manner. Additionally, the statement is confusing for viewers, as symptoms of PMS also occur regularly before a woman's menstrual cycle and the set of corresponding symptoms is identical to those associated with PMDD.

In this sense, it can be argued that PMDD, already classified as a form of disease mongering or disease branding, is continuing to be portrayed to consumers as a more serious, more severe condition that requires individual intervention. The intervention implied here is a woman speaking with her physician in order to obtain the prescription drug. Here, there is power in the ability to diagnose oneself with not just a set of symptoms (PMS) associated with a natural bodily occurrence, but with a medically recognized disorder that brings along with it the social power to associate a name with a disease, to define and frame a particular set of symptoms that incorporate the diseased state, and to identify socially what is normal and what is deviant, thereby creating a sense of further social order for the body (Foucault 1984; Jutel 2009; Rosenberg 2002). The pharmaceutical ideology that puts profit above patient understanding further perpetuates a system of self-diagnosis, as can be seen via the example of PMDD in the YAZ advertisement, where a message is distributed that celebrates the commodity while seamlessly appearing to put decisions about health into the hands of consumers. If the consumer does not take responsibility for their own health and participate in the promotional efforts provided by Bayer, then he or she has failed to be a "good" consumer (Ebeling 2011).

The advertisement continues by introducing a new character – a young, petite woman with short red hair. She is shown by herself in an upscale, yet bare, apartment, presumably in a city setting and it is evident that she has either recently moved in or is in the process of changing her home décor. The entire room is white, and she is shown climbing up a small ladder with a paint roller. As the camera pans, you can see that one of the walls is being painted a bright orange color. She glances at the camera while running one of her hands through her hair and smiles in a way that reveals she is proud of her ability to take ownership of her space. Not only is she independently renovating a portion of her domain, but she is doing so in a way that reflects youth, freedom, and vitality – the color she has chosen to paint her walls is bright and daring. She is portrayed as taking change into her own hands, which is something the YAZ brand accentuates throughout its one-minute ad. As we are shown this scene, the narrator continues:

> Yaz has a different type of hormone that, for some, may increase potassium too much – so don't take Yaz if you have kidney, liver, or adrenal disease because this could cause serious heart and health problems. Tell your doctor if you're on daily long-term treatment for chronic conditions like cardiovascular or inflammatory diseases. Serious risks include: blood clot, stroke, and heart attack. Smoking increases these risks, especially if you're over 35, so don't smoke on Yaz. Don't take the pill if you've had any of these, certain cancers, or could be pregnant. The pill does not protect against HIV or STDs (Bayer 2010).

As the narrator is describing the risk information and side effects associated with YAZ, two new characters are introduced – both are young women that are fashionably dressed, and they are shown from behind walking into a room that features dress forms (mannequin bodies) dressed in contemporary clothing. Neither of the young women are featured in professional clothing, consistent with the other women in the ad, but rather are wearing outfits that denote youth, comfort, and style – not business. This aligns with the YAZ brand, which is appealing to young women and their ability to express their individuality. None of the women featured in this advertisement are shown working under authority or in any position of answering to anyone else. Women are shown in the fashion industry, painting their own bedroom walls, and cutting their own hair, all signifying individuality, independence, and a carefree attitude toward life while simultaneously reaffirming the notion that these aspects all rely on having the perfect appearance. The commercial continues with one of the women carrying a dress form in her arms, and the camera then shows the two women fixing the dress on the mannequin after it has been placed among the other dress forms in the room. It is clear that both are proud of the dress they have clearly designed, and as they are perfectly situating it on the dress form, they look at one another and smile. They each intertwine their arms together almost as if to hold hands, signifying friendship and happiness between the two.

Next, the advertisement cuts back to the young blonde woman sitting in the backseat of the cab that has just pulled her hair down and changed her outfit. We are only shown a close-up of her face, which features a playful smile, and once again, she is running her fingers through her hair. Then, we are brought back to the woman that leaned back into a full bathtub while wearing her clothes, and she now has a jar of children's bubbles in her hand and is blowing bubbles directly at the camera while laughing. The last shot of the advertisement shows the Asian woman who has cut her own hair, as she playfully runs her hands through her hair (indicating the carefree, unconventional approach all of the women in the advertisement embody) and smiles at the camera. In all three of these instances, the commercial has brought us back full-circle, showing how each of the women shown in the opening scenes has not only taken control of her own life in some aspect, but we are shown the happiness that has resulted in each life after doing so. As these final scenes are shown, the narrator concludes with "ask your health care provider about YAZ" (Bayer 2010). The Bayer logo, YAZ logo, and YAZ slogan are all shown on the screen together as the commercial comes to a close, signifying that the most important message to take away from the advertisement is the brand name. The logo reads "beyond birth control," pointing to how YAZ is positioned to be more than just a birth control.

Bayer's use of "beyond birth control," in reality, has two meanings. First, YAZ can be marketed as being beyond just a birth control because the FDA has approved its additional uses for moderate acne and PMDD. Upon further inspection, though, it is clear that YAZ is being marketed as "being more" in the sense that its consumptions allows women to "do more" in terms of their lifestyle, freedom, independence, and happiness. Women are not only given the message that they can do more with YAZ, but that they can be more as well, by becoming more fashionable, assertive, daring, youthful, and fun in association with obtaining this product. Birth control advertisements, in particular, perpetuate the idea that women are in need of sexual protection while at the same time framing them as a threat to society if left uncontrolled, ultimately placing women in a position of responsibility for regulating sexual activity and pregnancy (Casper and Carpenter 2009). For example, the YAZ advertisement narrates the words "doing more" as a way to describe that the pill is not only effective at preventing pregnancy, but that it may also help treat moderate acne and PMDD (premenstrual dysphoric disorder) (Bayer 2010). "Doing more," however, serves as a representation of the prescription drug treating more conditions, but allows the consumer to associate with what more they can do, or achieve, once they obtain the birth control.

To situate the context of this particular advertisement even further, it is important to note that at the time this commercial aired, Bayer used multiple platforms (not just television) to promote these types of self-diagnosis and pseudo-agency in one's health. In 2010, the website for Yaz (which consumers are encouraged to visit with 22 seconds of this advertisement featuring text with the YAZ website) featured a "YAZ Body Diary," subtitled "Get with the Program!" where women were provided with a checklist for a self-diagnosis of PMDD, the personalized results of which could be printed (including the YAZ and Bayer labels on the page) and handed directly to one's physician (see Table 5.3).

The checklist itself presents multiple ambiguities, as some options feature opposing symptoms/experiences or multiple answers offered in one category. For example, the checklist asks the user to categorize whether she slept more, took naps, or found it hard to get up when intended, yet in the same category asks if she had trouble falling asleep or staying asleep (Ebeling 2011). The 2010 website was targeted to young women, with the home page featuring images of smiling, young women, all fashionable and engaging in activities ranging from applying makeup to playing the electric guitar (Ebeling 2011). Among the safety information for YAZ at the top of the webpage, there were also various tabs, labeled "The Works: Fashion & Style," and "Front Row: Hollywood Buzz," which led visitors to links of articles on the latest trends in fashion, beauty, and celebrity news. Each tab featured hypercommercialized forms of co-branding with other brands targeting female consumers, including cosmetics, high-end fashion designers, and women's magazines. The website for YAZ is another example of the ways

Table 5.3   2010 YAZ Website Body Diary Rating Scale for PMDD Titled "Get with the Program!"

Daily Record of Severity of Problems
Your rating on a scale from 0 to 5: (0: NOT AT ALL, 1: MINIMAL, 2: MILD, 3: MODERATE, 4: SEVERE, 5: EXTREME)

1. Felt depressed, sad, "down," or "blue" or felt hopeless; or felt worthless or guilty
2. Felt anxious, tense, "keyed up" or "on edge"
3. Had mood swings (i.e. suddenly feeling sad or tearful) or was sensitive to rejection or feelings were easily hurt
4. Felt angry or irritable
5. Had less interest in usual activities (work, school, friends, hobbies)
6. Had difficulty concentrating
7. Felt lethargic, tired, or fatigued; or had lack of energy
8. Had increased appetite or overate; or had cravings for specific foods
9. Slept more, took naps, found it hard to get up when intended; or had trouble getting to sleep or staying asleep
10. Felt overwhelmed or unable to cope; or felt out of control
11. Had breast tenderness, breast swelling; bloated sensation, weight gain, headache, or joint and muscle pain, or other physical symptoms
12. At work, school, home, or in daily routine, at least one of the problems noted above caused reduction of productivity or inefficiency
13. At least one of the problems noted above caused avoidance or less participation in hobbies or social activities

Note: Table created by Janelle Applequist.
Source: Adapted from the physician's report for the YAZ Body Diary. Copyright Jean Edicott, PhD and Wilma Harrison, MD; Ebeling, 2011.

in which Bayer not only further commodified its oral contraceptive, but how it integrated its branding with images, links, products, and cross-promotion that all position the patient as a consumer above all else. This is evidenced by the fact that Bayer separated (and continues to do so) its drug website according to two target audiences – the physician and the patient. "Physician information" is explicitly labeled and features drug safety information, side effects, and interaction warnings, all in line with the informative nature that DTCA proponents claim constitutes the industry's marketing efforts. On the other hand, the website is framed first and foremost as a form of promotional material, with patients being given the information that includes a clear "spin," advertising a product to particular audiences with additional imagery, content, and appeal that are conducive to consumer culture.

HEALTH ISSUES OCCURRING AFTER
ADVERTISEMENT AIRED IN 2010

In 2012 (two years after the advertisement used in this chapter aired), the FDA announced that YAZ carried a higher risk of blood clots than other pills, requiring new labels for the prescription drug (Corbett Dooren 2012). YAZ combines estrogen from the female body with its key ingredient, drospirenone, a synthetic form of progestin only found in prescription oral contraceptives YAZ, Yasmin, and Ocella (all manufactured by Bayer) (Emison 2011). Studies conducted by the FDA in 2012 found that serious, potentially fatal, side effects were linked to these contraceptives. The most serious risks associated with YAZ are its increased risks of heart attack, stroke, or pulmonary embolism. The FDA found that women who take oral contraceptives containing drospirenone are 74% more likely to suffer from blood clots than other women taking contraceptives without the ingredient (Post, 2011). While it is normal for the body to clot blood, YAZ was found to cause an abnormal level of clotting, increasing the risk of clotting in women by more than 600% (Emison 2011). The abnormal blood clots can break away from the blood vessel and travel into other parts of the body. If a blood clot lodges in the brain, it can result in a stroke. Blood clots lodging in the pulmonary artery (the artery that supplies blood to the lungs), can result in pulmonary embolism. If a blood clot blocks the flow of blood through the entire body, it can cause a heart attack. YAZ was also linked to deep vein thrombosis and gallbladder disease.

Rather than pulling the drug off the market, the FDA ordered that Bayer print new labels and prescription leaflet inserts for the drugs, which is why as of 2014 they are still accessible to consumers, yet still carry the same amount of risk (Emison 2011). The FDA issued a safety warning that encouraged women to discuss the risk of blood clotting associated with taking an oral contraceptive with their physician, but the warning also urged for them to discuss the benefits of taking birth control as well (Wallis 2012). Bayer has announced that, as of January 2014, more than 10,000 lawsuits have been filed against YAZ because of the side effects described above (Post 2011; Fleishman 2014). Bayer has also announced that, to date, more than 7,660 claims have been settled, totaling more than $1.6 billion in payouts to women having consumed the prescription drug (Fleishman 2014).

As Bayer continued to fight the negative publicity surrounding the health problems associated with taking YAZ, in 2011, they introduced a new drug, BeYaz. BeYaz is chemically identical to YAZ, but has added Folic Acid (Vitamin B-9), making it legal to market the drug as a new formula. Yet, BeYaz still contains the controversial synthetic progestin drospirenone. To date, if you visit the website for YAZ, both YAZ and BeYaz are marketed together. This means that Bayer arguably rolled out a nearly identical birth control pill, simply giving it a new name for consumers to associate with more positively, but carrying with it all the same side effects found previously with YAZ (Emison 2011).

Recall earlier discussions of pharmaceutical fetishism in chapter three. This book defines pharmaceutical fetishism as the commodification of brand-name pharmaceutical drugs, which, via advertising and promotional cultures, ignore large-scale production and for-profit motives of "big pharma" while simultaneously reiterating a brand discourse that offers individuals additionally constructed meanings and discourse which promote medicine as a cultural authority in health care and prescription drugs as having the capability to solve individual problems beyond those for which a medicine is scientifically intended. The concept of pharmaceutical fetishism relies upon the forms of pseudo-autonomy presented to consumers, namely through DTC advertisements. The YAZ advertisement analyzed in this chapter serves as an example of the ways in which the pharmaceutical industry celebrates the commodity that is the prescription drug, simultaneously giving less service to the potential harm associated with consumption of these products. By continuously reaffirming the positive aspects associated with YAZ, Bayer has performed a type of pharmaceutical fetishism that presents the oral contraceptive as having the ability to deliver much more than its intended uses.

By offering women a commercialized lens through which to view menstruation and contraception, pharmaceutical industries claim to offer women freedom associated with having more reproductive choices than condoms or diaphragms, yet this exchange rests on a growing dependence on the practitioners, medical institutions, and pharmaceutical industry that provides the tools (the pills) for this "freedom" (Tone 2012). By continuing to portray pharmaceuticals as products designed to assist women in "taking back

control" of their reproductive freedom, cultural messages that frame femininity as a hygiene crisis are perpetuated (Kissling 2006).

Arguably, the oral contraceptive sector is one that targets women at
a young age (in their early twenties) in an effort to suggest particular brands
and products that women will loyally use for the rest of their menstrual lives,
further explaining Bayer's efforts to so adamantly promote the YAZ brand
through its advertisements, website, and promotional materials. The "choice"
being presented here to women (in the sense that they can have shorter,
lighter periods if they obtain a particular birth control pill) is, in fact, a choice
that did not previously exist. Historically, menstruation was not a choice,
but rather a normal process associated with the female body that was meant
to be dealt with (Woods 2013). By being marketed as "doing more" in relation to treating moderate acne and PMDD in addition to acting as a form of
contraception, YAZ is marketed as a medical breakthrough that materially
and discursively transforms menstruation and contraception into personal
choices, subsequently circumventing any discussions about its cultural value
or inherent risks (Woods 2013).

A common theme used in DTCA is the empowerment of women associated
with the consumption of a particular drug, and the 2010 version of a broadcast
advertisement for YAZ is no exception. The advertisement kept reverting back
to the agency and independence associated with the brand, portraying women
in situations that emphasized their choice, freedom, and free spirits. While
associating empowerment as it relates to feminist agency is seemingly positive, once presented through a lens of commodification (as done in DTCA),
these portrayals offer little to no opportunities for women to transcend consumption patterns as an individual, inhibiting the messages of autonomy from
connecting to real, social relations (Riordan 2001). Rather than deconstructing empowerment as a separate category, it is important to recognize these
occurrences alongside other previously mentioned issues of representation
in these ads, in an effort to show that these categories do not operate outside
other processes of gendering or classing – thereby working "within a visual
economy that remains profoundly ageist and heteronormative" (Gill 2009,
137). The culmination of these portrayals aide in particular constructions of
health and patient autonomy. In this case, each category, or "code," serves as
a source of guidance for signification by audience members (MacRury 2009).
These codes transfer from advertisements to consumers as particular codes
for behavior, allowing individuals to negotiate their own meanings from a
textual material (MacRury 2009).

These postfeminist representations of what it means to be a woman over-
shadow that half of the YAZ advertisement is devoted to side effects, which
include stroke, blood clot, and death. These representations disproportionately
target women as making their role in reproduction more visible than men's,

while simultaneously selling the confusing alternative message that being responsible in preventing pregnancy does not have to mean being responsible in other forms of societal norms (Nathanson 1991). These findings suggest a gendered shift in the organization of YAZ and its brand, as sexualized and gendered representations of women aide in a pseudo-agency being sold to consumers. The subtext of the YAZ advertisement is that the natural processes of the female body get in the way of a woman's personal and social functioning, leaving it the woman's responsibility to treat the symptoms associated with menstruation, masking this responsibility as a form of self-empowerment (Greenslit 2006). This equates addressing contraception and/or treating PMDD with YAZ as a feminist act, when in fact, asking one's physician about YAZ is more of a consumerist act than anything else.

Chapter 6

Looking Forward

Health communication informs our understanding of current medical practice(s) and, in particular, provides information on the benefits and harms of medical interventions. The ways in which patients are represented in health care are too often left out of the equation, in part because it is difficult to quantify and reckon against biomedically defined outcomes. Nonetheless, patient-centered outcomes have in recent years become an important focus not just for research, but even more importantly for ongoing public conversations. Also important to our conceptions of health, disease, those affected by disease – and even those understood to be healthy – is the influence of the pharmaceutical industry. Pharmaceutical marketing depends on advertisements that portray patients; how such images are used reveals much about company strategies to, inter alia, increase product sales.

With such assumptions in mind, this book was designed to achieve several goals: (1) to replicate previous studies of DTCA, (2) to examine levels of medicalization and pharmaceuticalization within these ads and the potential resulting influence upon society, and (3) to apply elements of critical advertising studies to DTC advertisements, including the prevalence of what this project referred to as "pharmaceutical fetishism" in such ads (i.e. the portrayal of DTC advertisements to increase happiness or control over one's life and how this term relates to commodity fetishism; how prescription drugs are glorified as a form of positive consumption). These goals were engaged using several methods, including political economy, content analysis, and textual analysis.

DTCA in the United States has become one of the most influential sectors in terms of its profit-making ability and its impact on consumer decisions. No longer relying solely on physicians to suggest medications, the pharmaceutical industry continues to invest in the advertising sector to influence

119

what is undeniably a profitable industry: the pharmaceutical consumer. This book began by providing an overview of the historical evolution of drug advertising and its regulation, outlining the interconnected relationships present between government agencies and the corporations that disseminate these products and their subsequent marketing efforts. As noted earlier, widespread use of DTC advertisements, especially in broadcasting, did not occur until after the Modernization Act of 1997. After this time, social issues involving DTC advertisements – including issues of safety, physician-patient relationships, the power of big pharma, and, most central to this book, cultural definitions of good health and good life – began to be debated and studied.

Proponents for DTCA argue they have the ability to educate the public about health conditions and available treatments, essentially offering empowerment for individuals to become more involved in their health care (Holmer, 1999). Understandably, medicine and pharmaceutical options are areas that have the ability to confuse individuals, and pharmaceutical advertisements theoretically have the ability to educate individuals on possible health conditions and subsequent treatment options. Additionally, in an area that often can be overwhelming to individuals, these promotions may seem as offering "power to the powerless," giving them the information necessary to be more proactive in discussing health care options with physicians. However, a question this book sought to address is whether this is a false sense of power, ultimately creating a sense of pseudo-autonomy to turn consumers into patients via the process of pharmaceutical fetishism. Critics of DTCA claim that these advertisements mislead consumers, prompting them to want products they may not need or that may be more expensive than other remedies, such as simple lifestyle changes (Hollon 1999). Of course, advertisements do serve a useful purpose for consumers in that they provide information that can aide in educating one about features, use, other products, and competitive pricing. That being said, the main point of advertisements is to sell products, increasing a bottom line for profit-making potential, so the argument that an advertisement is meant to educate a consumer seems to conflict with capitalist interests.

Despite much solid content work on DTC advertisements, chapter two discussed that there were arguably still areas to be explored. Two such limitations were discussed: emphases on print DTC advertisements and a fairly circumscribed range of persuasive appeals in the ads. Another is the use of one method – in most cases, the method being quantitative in nature. Mixed-methods analyses are not common within this literature, most often utilizing either quantitative or qualitative approaches (Faerber and Kreling 2014; Frosch et al. 2007; Gooblar and Carpenter 2013; Kaphingst, Dejong, Rudd, and Daltroy 2004; Yang, Seo, Patel, and Sansgiry 2012). Quantitative research has a much larger presence (Faerber and Kreling 2014;

Frosch et al. 2007; Kaphingst, Dejong, Rudd, and Daltroy 2004; Yang, Seo, Patel, and Sansgiry 2012) and when qualitative frameworks are used, analyses are most often performed on a historical level, tracing the FDA's role in pharmaceutical advertising and presenting both sides of the "pharmaceutical advertising debate." Although highly important, few critical works on DTCA as presenting limited courses of health prevention have been published (Landau 2011; Quesinberry Stokes 2013).

Critical Advertising Studies served as the main theoretical foundation and an important trajectory for this work, which positioned the logic of the system of DTCA as one where consumers are molded into salespersons for prescriptions drugs, ultimately becoming the main sales force, as these advertisements become an intermediary between physicians and patients. Finally, this book argued for a triangulated approach to DTCA research.

This book found four major themes that are representative of the mixed-methods analyses chapters (four, five, and six). The first common theme features a continuation, and increase, of DTC advertisements undermining their informational function by emphasizing overwhelmingly positive outcomes of drug use, decreasing the educational content that focuses on health ailments particular drugs are designed to treat, and discouraging serious considerations of risk factors and other treatment options. Thus, as the pharmaceutical industry continues to claim that its advertising serves as a form of education for consumers regarding particular health ailments, this study shows that, in terms of the ability to have control in one's own life, the industry often emphasizes the product or the brand and its positive attributes more so than the corresponding health condition, the population at risk, alternative non-pharamaceutical techniques/treatments, and where to obtain more information about the condition.

The second major theme to result from this book involves the use of positive emotional appeals in DTC advertisements. Positive emotional appeals are continuing to be used in DTC advertisements since Frosch et al.'s original study, yet negative emotional appeals in the current dataset decreased considerably, highlighting how the pharmaceutical industry has attempted to persuade consumers to identify most with the positive, beneficial aspects of particular drugs. A common association with the use of positive emotional appeals in this study features perceived endurance and protection from other health risks. While only 12.4% of Frosch et al.'s (2007) sample featured characters that had increased endurance as a result of taking a medication, this study found that 72.2% of advertisements featured an increase in endurance and individual ability. The most common positive emotional appeal in the sample featured characters before and after they had consumed a medication, with an increase in the use of positive emotions and lifestyle portrayals shown after a character had obtained the drug. This signified an increase effort to positively associate their brand with a happier, healthier life. The majority of pharmaceutical advertisements in this study featured the narration of a medical disclaimer and/or presentation of side effects as a character was being shown only after consuming a prescription drug, portraying their positive experiences with drugs while the advertisements themselves are attempting to warn consumers of potentially harmful effects.

The third, and arguably most notable, theme found in this book is the practice of pharmaceutical advertisements explicitly utilizing advertising as a means of presenting prescription drugs as cures for more than just health conditions. Drugs are advertised in a way that presents them as having the added benefit of selling a particular lifestyle to individuals – one that emphasizes happiness, successful relationships, nuclear family activities, and personal fulfillment. Such ads, then, perpetuated the concept of commodity fetishism (Marx 1992) and the true social relations embedded in branded goods (such as industrial production contexts) are downplayed, while symbolically constructed consumption benefits are emphasized and, arguably, exaggerated. Thus, products appear to have value inherent in them, but the fact is that human beings themselves produce the additional value as enacted in a consumer culture. DTC advertisements enact commodity fetishism in a particular way, defined by this book as pharmaceutical fetishism, or the commodification of brand-name pharmaceutical drugs, which, via advertising and promotional cultures, ignore large-scale production and for-profit motives of "big pharma" while simultaneously reiterating a brand discourse that promotes medicine as a cultural authority in health care and prescription drugs as having the capability to solve individual problems beyond those for which a medicine is scientifically intended. The concept of pharmaceutical fetishism relies upon the forms of pseudo-autonomy presented to consumers, namely through DTC advertisements.

DTC advertisements present consumers with romanticized portrayals regarding what benefits a prescription drug can offer and ignoring other treatment options. Rather than relying merely on the medical benefits associated with a drug designed to treat a target condition, the industry of DTCA has permitted these commercials to include "additional benefits," usually by relying on the use of emotional appeals or presentations of scenarios of those in the ads who have used the drugs. This means that the culture of prescription drugs is being reproduced, potentially suggesting to consumers that they can obtain positive attributes beyond what can be corrected in the body – for example, advertisements for antidepressants often feature all relationships as significantly improving and seeming "perfect" as a result of consuming a medication, but this is a veiled representation of a serious mental health condition and the social challenges that come along with it. Similarly, the related concept of "disease mongering" was discussed in the chapter involving YAZ, which was sold as a skin condition as well as a form of birth control – all leading to a happier and fun-filled life, according to the ads. In order to benefit capitalistic endeavors, the culture of pharmaceuticals has evolved into one that promises much more than it can realistically deliver for consumers. As Rose (2007) has suggested, DTCA may be an aspect of medicalization and pharmaceuticalization that offer facile solutions to human needs of consumers. Furthermore, these solutions are often harmful, as they are presented to consumers in a way that leads them to believe that prescription drugs can remedy individual problems and fulfill personal desires. This can be described as a form of ideological appropriation, as the industry that exists to expand understandings of health is the very industry that creates false needs in a consumer-driven market (Abraham 2010).

Finally, the fourth major theme to result from this book is the ways in which DTC advertisements perpetuate normalized conceptions of particular representations, featuring characters that portray stereotypical gender roles, youthfulness even in cases of being older, heteronormative relationships, familial relationships as being central to health, and patients as being autonomous from their physicians. For example, women are featured in advertisements as being empowered. Yet, while associating empowerment as it relates to feminist agency is seemingly positive, once presented through a lens of commodification (as done in DTCA), these portrayals offer little to no opportunities for women to transcend consumption patterns as an individual, inhibiting the messages of autonomy from connecting to real, social relations (Riordan 2001). Rather than deconstructing empowerment as a separate category, it is important to recognize these occurrences alongside other previously mentioned issues of representation in these ads, in an effort to show that these categories do not operate outside other processes of gendering or classing – thereby working "within a visual economy that remains profoundly ageist and heteronormative" (Gill 2009, 137). The culmination of these portrayals aide in particular constructions of health and patient autonomy, but ones that ultimately benefit large drug companies. In this case, each category, or "code," serves as a source of guidance for signification by – and even of – audience members (MacRury 2009).

The limitations of this book are predominantly associated with the analysis chapters (four and five). Given the large sample size of the analyses conducted for this project, and the high number of variables used, it is possible that important interpretations, findings, or themes were not addressed in the final write-up. That being said, this sample could be useful for future work that would like to take a more focused approach to DTC advertisements (for example, a study could entirely focus on representations of gender). Also, it would be useful for research to contextualize the findings of this book by repeating the analyses using a more current dataset.

A second limitation to this book is its use of primetime television programming. Had a niche network (such as ESPN or Lifetime) been used, perhaps more context could have been provided regarding target audiences and issues of representation found in these advertisements.

Of course, as a text-based study, assumptions are made about how audiences may interpret the symbolic tendencies of these ad-texts. As noted earlier, advertising involves an often complex set of semiotic codes about the brand, people, society and abstract concepts such as happiness and good health. These codes transfer from advertisements to consumers as particular codes for behavior, allowing individuals to negotiate their own meanings from a textual material (MacRury 2009). Audience-based studies looking at how audiences make meaning of definitions of health, heath authorities, and the good life would be valuable additions to text-oriented research such as this one.

While this book serves to supplement Western interpretations of health communication, future work would benefit by bridging internationally, focusing on the ways in which DTCA impacts culture, health, and regulatory issues in New Zealand, the only other industrialized nation in the world that permits these types of advertisements on television. This project is concluding by proposing international communications research that analyzes data on DTC advertisements from a larger scale, including the United States and New Zealand. As two schools of thought have emerged from studying the presence of these advertisements, as this book has shown, pharmaceutical advertisements have the potential to educate patients and promote informed choice, however, ads in the United States rely primarily on emotional appeals while providing often complex drug information that is difficult for consumers to understand. In order to understand the ways in which patients are being framed by the prescription drug market, it is necessary to gain a larger perspective on this issue, meaning that data from New Zealand must be considered alongside that from the United States. Although previous research has indicated some similarities and differences in the pharmaceutical advertisements of each nation, more work is required to understand the potential implications of pharmaceutical advertising from an international perspective. Simply stated, the content and context of these advertisements require further analysis in order to understand how the pharmaceutical industry views its patients on an international level. Becoming part of the culture in order to gain social context and insight as to how the citizens of New Zealand feel about DTC advertisements, and their effectiveness, is necessary. Additionally, future research should nuance the presentation of this book's political economic (industry-focused)/public relations framework. Namely, research should more explicitly understand and the set of relations existent in the pharmaceutical industry that reflects greater complexities and ambiguities.

By incorporating a cultural studies perspective more incorporative of scholars such as Giddens and Bourdieu, institutional theories of organization can be utilized alongside descriptive case studies in order to address the modalities surrounding the microsocial engagements of the pharmaceutical industry and its practices that more fully illuminates their relationships to DTCA and subsequent successes beyond just the ownership/corporate protocol previously described. By utilizing synergies, social relationships, and networking present within the pharmaceutical advertising industry, cultural studies scholarship could benefit from the influences that these connections have on larger social conceptions of health care and what it means for one to be deemed as "ill" or "healthy."

In regard to the quantitative portion of this study, future work should focus more on niche channels (e.g. Lifetime, ESPN, etc.) that feature pharmaceutical advertisements, as doing so would lend a different focus about very specific target audiences, ultimately leading to more descriptive analyses of patient representation. Future research could also benefit from further analyses of this data. This book considered content analyses, but did not address statistical significance of the findings, meaning that future research could use Chi Square analyses (perhaps using meta-analyses to examine data across studies) to show the ways in which trends have become more pronounced over time.

A discussion, and possible future research, regarding more normative approaches to patient education surrounding the subject of DTCA is necessary. Specifically, the concept of pharmaceutical fetishism is important not only for the academic audience to understand, but arguably even more so for patients. The results of this book, and accompanying discussions found within it, offer important implications for the ways in which media literacy is a crucial and important factor in helping to educate patients on pharmaceutical advertising culture and its selective, inflated – and sometimes even false – promises. For an individual who is not familiar with the nuances of Critical Advertising Studies, pharmaceutical fetishism may seem like a daunting concept. Using important foundations of media literacy, pharmaceutical fetishism should be defined for patients as pharmaceutical advertisements raising expectations too high regarding the efficacy of a prescription drug. Additionally, these advertisements promise viewers a happy (or happier) life, potentially leading to greater levels of unhappiness once it is realized that prescription drugs themselves cannot deliver such an idealized lifestyle. Media literacy could be a helpful approach in aiming to correct the problematic nature of DTCA, and it is important that future research investigates how patients could best understand what is at stake for their health care and even their overall life satisfaction when viewing these types of advertisements.

Finally, it is vital that research places these advertisements within a larger historical and theoretical context corresponding to their country and culture, as doing so can help to understand how medical knowledge has adapted over the years to position market forces of health care. These discussions have the potential to shed light on broader, safer alternatives that could benefit the ways we think of patients locally, nationally, and internationally. Previous research has acknowledged the importance of understanding how patients are represented, and in order for health communication research to serve as a form of patient advocacy, it is crucial that future studies continue to investigate how DTCA is most currently portraying the role of the patient within the larger context of the pharmaceutical industry. Ultimately, these discussions can lead to a greater understanding of national and international health care by extending how the logics of medical advertising may or may not be effective as related to cultural attributes, cultural policies, and various consumer identities.

Bibliography

Abbott Laboratories. "Trilipix," CBS. Television advertisement, aired 8 February 2010.

Abel, Gregory A., Stephanie J. Lee, and Jane C. Weeks. "Direct-to-consumer advertising in oncology: A content analysis of print media," *Journal of Clinical Oncology* 25, no. 10 (2007): 1267–1271, doi: 10.1634/theoncologist.11-2-217.

Abraham, John. "Partial progress: Governing the pharmaceutical industry and the NHS, 1948–2008," *Journal of Health, Politics, Law and Policy* 34 (2009): 931–977, doi: 10.1215/03616878-2009-032.

Abraham, John. "Pharmaceuticalization of society in context: Theoretical, empirical and health dimensions," *Sociology* 44, no. 4 (2010): 603–622, doi: 10.1177/0038038510369368.

Anderson, Paul J. "Study measures DTC impact," *Pharmaceutical Executive* 23, no. 8 (2003): 18.

Angell, Marcia. *The Truth About Drug Companies: How they Deceive Us and What to Do About It.* New York: Random House, 2004.

Arney, Jennifer K., and Benjamin Lewin. "Models of physician-patient relationships in pharmaceutical direct-to-consumer advertising and consumer interviews," *Qualitative Health Research* 23, no. 7 (2013): 937–950, doi: 10.1177/1049732313487801.

Arnold, Matthew. "Saatchi & Saatchi healthcare advertising," *Medical Marketing and Media* 44, no. 7 (2009): 152–153.

Arnould, Eric J., and Craig J. Thompson. "Consumer culture theory (CCT): Twenty years of research," *Journal of Consumer Research* 31 (2005): 868–882, doi: 10.1086/426626.

Baglia, Jay. *The Viagra AdVenture: Masculinity, Media and the Performance of Sexual Health.* New York: Peter Lang, 2005.

Banerjee, Mousumi, Michelle Capozzoli, Laura McSweeney, and Debajyoti Sinha. "Beyond kappa: A review of interrater agreement measures," *The Canadian Journal of Statistics* 27 (1999): 3–23, doi: 10.2307/3315487.

Bandura, Albert. "Social cognitive theory of mass communication," In *Media Effects: Advances in Theory and Research*, edited by Jennings Bryant and Doli Zillmann, 121–153. Mahwah: Lawrence Erlbaum, 2002.

Barker, Kristin K. "Listening to Lyrica: Contested illnesses and pharmaceutical determinism," *Social Science & Medicine* 73 (2011): 833–842, doi: 10.1016/j.socscimed.2011.05.055.

Bayer. "Yaz." ABC. Television advertisement, aired 15 March 2010.

Bell, Robert A., Richard L. Kravitz, and Michael S. Wilkes. "Direct-to-consumer prescription drug advertising, 1989-1998," *The Journal of Family Practice* 49, no. 4 (1999): 329–335.

Bell, Robert A., Richard L. Kravitz, and Michael S. Wilkes. "The educational value of consumer-targeted prescription drug advertising," *Journal of Family Practice* 49, no. 12 (2000): 1092–1098.

Bennett, Andy. *Culture and Everyday Life*. London: Sage Publications, 2005.

Beltramini, Richard F. "Consumer believability of information in direct-to-consumer (DTC) advertising of prescription drugs," *Journal of Business Ethics* 63 (2006): 333–343, doi: 10.1007/s10551-005-4711-2.

Berelson, Bernard. *Content Analysis in Communication Research*. Glencoe: Free Press, 1952.

Bergner, Kai N., Tomas Falk, Daniel Heinrich, and Jörg A. Hölzing. (2013). "The effects of DTCA on patient compliance," *International Journal of Pharmaceutical and Healthcare Marketing* 7, no. 4 (2013): 391-409.

Bernard, H. Russell. *Research Methods in Anthropology: Qualitative and Quantitative Approaches*. Lanham: AltaMira Press, 2006.

Bernard, Stan, and Janet Wells. "Blockbuster 2.0: Eight ways to follow that leader," *Pharmaceutical Executive*, June 9, 2015, http://www.pharmexec.com/blockbuster-20-eight-ways-follow-leader.

Bernstein, Marver H. *Regulating Business by Independent Commission*. Princeton: Princeton University Press, 1955.

Bernstein, David S. "Med school drug pushers: How scientists are selling out to drug companies," *The Phoenix*, January 28 2010, http://thephoenix.com/boston/news/8920-med-school-drug-pushers/.

Bhatia, Subhash C., and Bhatia, Shashi K. (2002). "Diagnosis and treatment of premenstrual dysphoric disorder," *American Family Physician* 66, no. 7 (2002): 1239–1249.

Bittar, Christine. "Act two from the Purple Pill," *Brandweek* 45, no. 36 (2004): M54–M57.

Bogard, Cynthia J. "Claimsmakers and contexts in early constructions of homelessness: A comparison of New York City and Washington, D.C.," *Symbolic Interaction* 24 (2001): 425–454, doi: 10.1525/si.2001.24.4.425.

Bowles, Samuel, and Richard Edwards. *Understanding Capitalism*. New York: HarperCollins, 1993.

Breazeale, Kenon. "In spite of women: Esquire magazine and the construction of the male consumer," *Signs* 20 (1994): 1–22.

Brinberg, David, and Louise H. Kidder. *Forms of Validity in Research*. San Francisco: Jossey-Bass, 1982.

Bristol-Myers Squibb Co. 2010a. "Plavix Version One." ABC. Aired 2 May 2010.

Bristol-Myers Squibb Co. 2010b. "Plavix Version Two." CBS. Aired 23 April 2010.

Bristol-Myers Squibb Co. 2010c. "Abilify Version One." FOX. Aired 10 February 2010.

Bristol-Myers Squibb Co. 2010d. "Abilify Version Two." ABC. Aired 13 April 2010.

Brownfield, Erica D., Jay M. Bernhardt, Jennifer L. Phan, Mark V. Williams, and Ruth M. Parker. "Direct-to-consumer drug advertisements on network television: An exploration of quantity, frequency, and placement," *Journal of Health Communication* 9, no. 6 (2014): 491–497, doi: 10.1080/10810730490523115.

Bryman, Alan, and Robert G. Burgess. *Analyzing Qualitative Data*. London: Routledge, 1994.

Budd, Mike, Steve Craig, and Clay Steinman. *Consuming Environments: Television and Commercial Culture*. New Brunswick: Rutgers University Press, 1999.

Burn, Shawn Megan. *The Social Psychology of Gender*. New York: McGraw-Hill, 1996.

Campbell, Margaret C., and Kevin Lane Keller. "Brand familiarity and advertising repetition effects," *Journal of Consumer Research* 30, no. 2 (2003): 292–304, doi: 10.1086/376800

Calfee, John E. "Public policy issues in direct-to-consumer advertising of prescription drugs," *Journal of Public Policy & Marketing* 21, no. 2 (2002): 174–193, doi: 10.1509/jppm.21.2.174.17580.

Carlson, Matt. "Boardroom brothers: Interlocking directorates indicate media's corporate ties," *Extra!* September (2001): 18–19.

Carmines, Edward G., and Richard A. Zeller. *Reliability and Validity Assessment*. Thousand Oaks: Sage, 1979.

Carney, T. F. "Content analysis: A review essay," *Historical Methods* 4, no. 2 (1971): 52–61. doi: 10.1080/00182494.1971.10593939.

Carrigan, Marlyn, and Isabelle Szmigin. "Advertising and older consumers: Image and ageism," *Business Ethics: A European Review* 9, no. 1 (2002): 42–50, doi: 10.1111/1467-8608.00168.

Casper, Monica J., and Laura M. Carpenter. "Sex, Drugs, and Politics: The HPV Vaccine for Cervical Cancer." In *Pharmaceuticals and Society: Critical Discourses and Debates*, edited by Simon J. Williams, Jonathan Gabe, and Peter Davis, 71–84. Malden: Wiley-Blackwell, 2009.

Chambers, Derek, and Susan Thompson. "Empowerment and its application in health promotion in acute care settings: Nurses' perceptions," Journal of Advanced Nursing 65 (2008): 130–138, doi: 10.1111/j.1365-2648.2008.04851.x.

Chaney, David. "Creating memories: Some Images of Ageing in Mass Tourism." In *Images of Ageing: Cultural Representations of Later Life*, edited by Mike Featherstone and Andrew Wernick, 209–224. London: Routledge, 1995.

Chandler, Jon, and Mike Owen. "Pharmaceuticals: The new brand arena," *International Journal of Marketing Research* 44, Q4 (2002).

Charmaz, K. *Good Days, Bad Days: The Self in Chronic Illness and Time*. New Brunswick: Rutgers University Press, 1991.

Charmaz, Kathy. *Constructing Grounded Theory: A Practical Guide Through Qualitative Analysis*. Thousand Oaks: Sage Publications, 2006.

Chimonas, Susan, and Jermone Kassiser. "No more free drug samples?" *PLoS Medicine* 6, no. 5 (2009), doi: 10.1371/journal.pmed.1000074.

Clarke, Adele E., Janet K. Shim, Laura Mamo, Jennifer Ruth Fosket, and Jennifer R. Fishman. "Biomedicalization: Technoscientific transformations of health, illness, and US biomedicine," *American Sociological Review* 68 (2003): 161–194.

Cohen, Jacob. "A coefficient of agreement for nominal scales," *Educational and Psychological Measurement* 20 (1960): 37–46, doi: 10.1177/001316446002000104.

Cohen, Jacob. "Weighted kappa: Nominal scale agreement with provision for scaled disagreement of partial credit," *Psychological Bulletin* 70 (1968): 213–220.

Comstock, George A., Susan Lloyd-Jones, and Eli A. Rubinstein. *Television and Social Behavior: Reports and Papers*. Rockville: National Institute of Mental Health, 1972.

Conrad, Peter. *The Medicalization of Society: On the Transformation of Human Conditions into Treatable Disorders*. Baltimore: Johns Hopkins University Press, 2007.

Conrad, Peter, and Valerie Leiter. "Medicalization, markets and consumers," *Journal of Health and Social Behavior* 45 (2004): 158–176.

Conrad, Peter, and Valerie Leiter. "From lydia pinkham to queen levitra: Direct-to-consumer advertising and medicalization," *Sociology of Health and Illness* 30 (2008): 825–838, doi: 10.1111/j.1467-9566.2008.01092.x.

Corbett Dooren, Jennifer. Clotting Risks for Yaz Pill, *Wall Street Journal*, April 10 2012, http://www.wsj.com/articles/SB10001424052702304587704577336113766301968.

Crockett, David. "Marketing blackness: How advertisers use race to sell products," *Journal of Consumer Culture* 8, no. 2 (2008): 245–268, doi: 10.1177/1469540508090088.

Cross, Gary. "Origins of modern consumption: Advertising, new goods, and a new generation, 1890–1930." In *The Routledge Companion to Advertising and Promotional Culture,* edited by Emily West and Matthew P. McAllister, 11–23. New York: Routledge, 2013.

DeLorme, Denise E., Jisu Huh, and Leonard N. Reid. "'Others are influenced, but not me': Older adults' perceptions of DTC prescription drug advertising effects," *Journal of Aging Studies* 21 (2007): 135–151.

Department of Health and Human Services. Food and Drug Administration *21 CFR Part 202*. Federal Register 75, no. 59 15376–15387. Washington, D.C.: United States Government Printing Office, 2010.

Desselle, Shane Paul, and Ratendar Aparasu. "Attitudinal dimensions that determinepharmacists' decisions to support DTCA of prescription medication," *Therapeutic Innovation & Regulatory Science* 34 (2000): 103–114.

Dewey, M. E. "Coefficients of agreement," *The British Journal of Psychiatry* 143, no. 5 (1983): 487–489, doi: 10.1192/bjp.143.5.487.

Dey, Ian. *Qualitative Data Analysis: A User-Friendly Guide for Social Scientists*. London: Routledge, 1993

Dickinson, Greg. "Selling democracy: Consumer culture and citizenship in the wake of September 11," *The Southern Communication Journal* 70, no. 4 (2005): 271–284.

Dines, Gail, and Jean McMahon Humez. *Gender, Race, and Class in Media: A Critical Reader*. 4th edition. Thousand Oaks: Sage, 2015.

Dow, Bonnie. "*Ellen*, Television, and the Politics of Gay and Lesbian Visibility," Critical Studies in Media Communication 18, no. 2 (2001): 123–140. doi: 10.1080/07393180128077

Durham-Humphrey Amendment, U.S. Stat. 65 (1951), § 648.

Ebeling, Mary. "'Get with the program!': Pharmaceutical marketing, symptom checklists and self-diagnosis," Social Science & Medicine 73, no. 6 (2011): 825–832, doi: 10.1016/j.socscimed.2011.05.054.

Eli Lilly. 2010a. "Cymbalta." ABC. Aired 5 April 2010.

Eli Lilly. 2010b. "Cialis Version One." CBS. Aired 15 February 2010.

Eli Lilly. 2010c. "Cialis Version Two." CBS. Aired 21 April 2010.

Elliott, Carl. The Drug Pushers. *The Atlantic*, April 2006, http://www.theatlantic.com/magazine/archive/2006/04/the-drug-pushers/304714/.

Elliott, Carl. *White Coat, Black Hat: Adventures on the Dark Side of Medicine*. Boston: Beacon, 2010a.

Elliott, Carl. How to Brand a Disease—and Sell a Cure, *CNN*, October 11 2010b, http://www.cnn.com/2010/OPINION/10/11/elliott.branding.disease/.

Ellis, Lee. *Research Methods in the Social Sciences*. Madison: Brown & Benchmark, 1994.

Emison, Brett. Bayer's Beyaz Birth Control Pill: New Name, Same Side Effects, *The Legal Examiner*, January 20 2011, http://kansascity.legalexaminer.com/fda-prescription-drugs/bayers-beyaz-birth-control-pill-new-name-same-side-effects/.

Engelhardt, Tristram H. *The Foundations of Bioethics*. 2nd edition. New York: Oxford University Press, 1986.

Erlandson, David A., Edward L. Harris, Barbara L. Skipper, and Steve D. Allen. *Doing Naturalistic Inquiry: A Guide to Methods*. Newbury Park: Sage, 1993.

Faerber, Adrienne E., and David H. Kreling. "Content analysis of false and misleading claims in television advertising for prescription and nonprescription drugs," *Journal of General Internal Medicine* 29, no. 1 (2014): 110-118, doi: 10.1080/10810730490523115.

Farris, Paul W., and William L. Wilkie. "Marketing scholars' roles in the policy arena: An opportunity for discourse on direct-to-consumer advertising," *Journal of Public Policy & Marketing* 24, spring (2005): 1–2.

Finfgeld, Deborah L. "Empowerment of individuals with enduring mental health problems: Results from concept analyses and qualitative investigations," *Nursing Science* 27 (2004): 44-52.

Fiske, John, and John Hartley. *Reading Television*. London: Methuen, 1978.

Fleishman, Wendy. "Is YAZ Safe for Me?" 2014, http://www.lieffcabraser.com/blog/2014/01/is-Yaz-safe-for-me.shtml.

Fornell, Claes, and David F. Larcker. "Evaluating structural equation models with unobservable variable and measurement error," *Journal of Marketing Research* 18, February (1981): 39–50.

Food and Drug Administration Modernization Act, 21 U.S.C. § 301 (1997).

"Fortune 500: 2012," Fortune, May, 2013, http://money.cnn.com/magazines/fortune/fortune500/2013/full_list/.

Foucault, Michel. "The politics of health in the eighteenth century," In *The Foucault Reader*, edited by Paul Rabinow. New York: Pantheon, 1984.

Foucault, Michael. "The subject of power," In *Michael Foucault: Structuralism and Hermeneutics*, edited by Hubert L. Dreyfus and Paul Rabinow. Chicago: Chicago University Press, 1983.

Foucault, Michel. *The Birth of the Clinic: An Archaeology of Medical Perception*. New York: Pantheon Books, 1994.

Fox, Nick J., and Katie J. Ward. "Pharma in the bedroom...and the kitchen...the pharmaceuticalisation of daily life," In *Pharmaceuticals and Society*, edited by Simon J. Williams, Jonathan Gabe, and Peter Davis, 41–53. Chichester: Wiley-Blackwell, 2009.

Frey, Lawrence R., Carl H. Botan, and Gary L. Kreps. *Investigating Communication: An Introduction to Research Methods*. 2nd edition. Boston: Allyn & Bacon, 2000.

Friedan, Betty. *The Feminine Mystique*. New York: W. W. Norton & Company, 1963.

Frosch, Dominick L., and Robert M. Kaplan. "Shared decision making in clinical medicine: Past research and future directions," *American Journal of Preventive Medicine* 17, no. 4 (1999): 285–294.

Frosch, Dominick L., Patrick M. Krueger, Robert C. Hornik, Peter F. Cronholm, and Frances K. Barg. "Creating demand for prescription drugs: A content analysis of television direct-to-consumer advertising," *Annals of Family Medicine* 5, no. 1 (2007): 6–13, doi: 10.1370/afm.611.

Fugh-Berman, Adriane, and Shahram Ahari. "Following the script: How drug reps makefriends and influence doctors," *PLoS Medicine* 4, no. 4 (2007), doi:10.1371/journal.pmed.0040150.

Fuqua, Joy V. *Prescription TV: Therapeutic Discourse in the Hospital and at Home*. Durham: Duke University Press, 2012.

Gatignon, Hubert, and Thomas S. Robertson. "A propositional inventory for new diffusion research," *Journal of Consumer Research* 11, no. 3 (1985): 849–867.

Gellad, Ziad F., and Kenneth W. Lyles. "Direct-to-consumer advertising of pharmaceuticals," *The American Journal of Medicine* 120 (2007): 475–480, doi: 10.1016/j.amjmed.2006.09.030.

Germeni, Evi, Grazia Orizio, Kent Nakamoto, Martha Wunsch, and P. J. Schulz. "American physician perceptions of direct-to-consumer advertising: A qualitative study," *Journal of Communication in Healthcare* 6, no. 2 (2013): 135–141, doi: 10.1179/1753807613Y.0000000034.

Gilbert, David, Tom Walley, and Bill New. "Lifestyle medicines," *British Medical Journal* 321 (2000): 1341–1344.

Gill, Rosalind C. "Beyond the 'sexualization of culture' thesis: An intersectional analysis of 'sixpacks,' 'midriffs,' and 'hot lesbians' in advertising," *Sexualities* 12, no. 2 (2009): 137–160, doi: 10.1177/1363460708100916.

Glaser, Barney G. *Theoretical Sensitivity: Advances in the Methodology of Grounded Theory*. Mill Valley: Sociology Press, 1978.

Glaser, Barney G., and Anselm L. Strauss. *The Discovery of Grounded Theory: Strategies for Qualitative Research*. Chicago: Aldine, 1967.

GlaxoSmithKline. "Advair Version One." ABC. Television advertisement, aired 12 April 2010a.

GlaxoSmithKline. "Advair Version Two," CBS. Television advertisement, aired 3 February 2010b.

Goffman, Erving. *Gender Advertisements*. New York: Harper and Row, 1979.

Goldberg, Michele, and Bob Davenport. "In sales we trust," *Pharmaceutical Executive*, 2005, http://www.pharmexec.com.

Goldman, Robert. *Reading Ads Socially*. New York: Routledge, 1992.

Goldman, Robert, and Stephen Papson. *Sign Wars: The Cluttered Landscape of Advertising*. New York: Guilford Press, 1996.

Gooblar, Jonathan, and Brian D. Carpenter. "Print advertisements for Alzheimer's disease drugs: Informational and transformational features," *American Journal of Alzheimer's Disease & Other Dementias* 28, no. 4 (2013): 355–362, doi: 10.1177/1533317513488912.

Gray, Judy H., and Iain L. Densten. "Integrating quantitative and qualitative analysis using latent and manifest variables," *Quality & Quantity* 32 (1998): 419–431, doi: 10.1023/A:1004357719066.

Greenslit, Nathan. "Depression and consumption: Psychopharmaceuticals, branding, and new identity practices," *Culture, Medicine and Psychiatry* 29 (2005): 477–501, doi: 10.1007/s11013-006-9005-3.

Gross, Gregory, and Robert Blundo. "Viagra: Medical technology constructing aging masculinity," *Journal of Sociology and Social Welfare* 32, no. 1 (2005): 85–97.

Haas, Jennifer S., Kathryn A. Phillips, Eric P. Gerstenberger, and Andrew C. Serger. "Potential savings from substituting generic drugs for brand-name drugs: Medical expenditure panel survey," *Archives of Internal Medicine* 142, no. 11 (2005): 891–897.

Hains, Rebecca C. "Power feminism, mediated: Girl power and the commercial politics of change," *Women's Studies in Communication* 32, no. 1 (2009): 89–113.

Hair, Joseph F., Ronald E. Anderson, Rolph E. Tatham, and William C. Black. *Multivariate Data Analysis*. 5th edition. Upper Saddle River: Prentice Hall, 1998.

Heinrich, Janet. *Prescription Drugs: FDA Oversight of Direct-to-Consumer Advertising has Limitations*. Washington: U.S. General Accounting Office, 2002, 1–53.

Herper, Matthew. "The best-selling drugs in America," *Forbes*, April 19, 2011, http://www.forbes.com/sites/matthewherper/2011/04/19/the-best-selling-drugs-in- america/2/.

Hollon, Matthew F. "Direct-to-consumer marketing of prescription drugs: Creating consumer demand," *Journal of the American Medical Association* 281, no. 4 (1999): 382–384.

Hollows, Joanne. "Feeling like a domestic goddess: Postfeminism and cooking," *European Journal of Cultural Studies* 6, no. 2 (2003): 179–202, doi: 10.1177/13675 49403006002003.

Holmer, Alan F. "Direct-to-consumer prescription drug advertising builds bridges between patients and physicians," *Journal of the American Medical Association* 281, no. 4 (1999): 380–382.

Holmer, Alan F. "Direct-to-consumer advertising--strengthening our health care system," *New England Journal of Medicine* 346, no. 7 (2002): 526–528, doi: 10.1056/NEJM200202143460714.

Holmes, Erin R., and Shane P. Desselle. "Evaluating the balance of persuasive and informative content within product-specific print direct-to-consumer ads," *Drug Information Journal* 38, no. 1 (2004): 83–98.

Holsti, Ole R. *Content Analysis for the Social Sciences and Humanities*. Reading: Addison-Wesley, 1969.

Horkheimer, Max, and Theodor W. Adorno. *Dialectic of Enlightenment*. New York: Herder and Herder, 1972.

Horwitz, Allan V. *The Irony of Regulatory Reform: The Deregulation of American Telecommunications*. Oxford: Oxford University Press, 1989.

Horwitz, Allan V., and Jerome C. Wakefield. "The medicalization of sadness," *Salute e Società* 8 (2009): 49–66.

Hyojin, Kim, and Lee Chunsik. "Differential effects of fear-eliciting DTCA on elaboration, perceived endorser credibility, and attitudes," *International Journal of Pharmaceutical and Healthcare Marketing* 6, no. 1 (2012): 4–22, doi: http://dx.doi.org/10.1108/17506121211216860.

Hunt, Michie I. "Prescription drugs and intellectual property protection." National Institute for Health Care Management, 2000.

Illich, Ivan. *Medical Nemesis: The Expropriation of Health*. London: Marion Boyars Publisher Ltd., 1973.

Jack, Andrew. "Bayer rapped for medicine tweets," *The Financial Times*, August 16, 2011.

Janssen Pharmaceuticals. "Simponi." NBC. Television advertisement, aired 20 March 2010.

Jennewein, Klaus, Thomas Durand, and Alexander Gerybadze. "When brands complement patients in securing the returns from technological innovation: The case of Bayer aspirin," *International Management* 14, no. 3 (2010): 73–86, doi: 10.7202/044294ar.

Jhally, Sut, and Bill Livant. "The valorization of consciousness: The political economy of symbolism," In *The Codes of Advertising: Fetishism and the Political Economy of Meaning in the Consumer Society*, edited by Sut Jhally, 64–121. New York: Routledge,1990.

Jhally, Sut. *The Codes of Advertising: Fetishism and the Political Economy of Meaning in the Consumer Society*. New York: Routledge, 1990.

Jordan, Amy, Dale Kunkel, Jennifer Manganello, and Martin Fishbein. *Media Messages and Public Health: A Decisions Approach to Content Analysis*. New York: Routledge, 2009.

Jutel, Annemaire. "Sociology of diagnosis: A preliminary review," *Sociology of Health & Illness* 31, no. 2 (2009): 278–299, doi: 10.1111/j.1467-9566.2008.01152.x.

Kantar Media. *Pharmaceutical Marketing—white paper*. New York: Ad Age, 2011.

Kaphingst, Kimberly A., William Dejong, Rima E. Rudd, and Lawren H. Daltroy. "A content analysis of direct-to-consumer television prescription drug advertisements," *Journal of Health Communication* 9 (2004): 515–528, doi: 10.1080/10810730490882586.

Kellner, Douglas M., and Meenakshi Gigi Durham. "Introduction: Adventures in media and cultural studies." In *Media and Cultural Studies: Key Works.* 2nd edition, edited by Douglas M. Kellner and Meenakshi Gigi Durham, 1–23. Malden: Wiley-Blackwell, 2012.

Kenneth, Kaitlin, and Joseph A. DiMassi. "Measuring the pace of drug development in the user fee era," *Drug Information Journal* 34 (2000): 673–680.

Kim, James H., and Anthony R. Scialli. "Thalidomide: The tragedy of birth defects and the effective treatment of disease," *Toxicological Sciences* 122 (2011): 1–6, doi: 10.1093/toxsci/kfr088.

Kissling, Elizabeth A. *Capitalizing on the Curse: The Business of Menstruation.* Boulder: Lynne Rienne, 2006.

Klein, Naomi. *No Logo.* London: HarperCollins, 2000.

Kotler, Philip, and Kevin Lane Keller. *Marketing Management.* Englewood Cliffs: Pearson Prentice Hall, 2006.

Kravitz, Richard L., Ronald M. Epstein, Mitchell D. Feldman, Carol E. Franz, and Rahman Azari. "Influence of patients' requests for direct-to-consumer advertised antidepressants: A randomized controlled trial," *Journal of the American Medical Association* 293 (2005): 1995–2002, doi: 10.1001/jama.293.16.1995.

Krippendorff, Klaus. "Reliability in content analysis: Some common misconceptions and recommendations," *Human Communication Research* 30, no. 3 (2004): 411–433, doi: 10.1111/j.1468-2958.2004.tb00738.x.

Kumar, Pankaj, and Ron Brand. "Detailing Gets Personal," *Pharmaceutical Executive*, 2003. http://www.pharmexec.com/pharmexec/article/articleDetail.jsp?id=64071.

Landau, Jamie. "Women will get cancer: Visual and verbal presence in a pharmaceutical advertising campaign about HPV," *Argumentation & Advocacy* 48 (2011): 39–54.

Laverack, Glenn. *Public Health: Power, Empowerment and Professional Practice.* 2nd edition. New York: Palgrave Macmillan, 2009.

Light, Donald W., and Joel R. Lexchin. "Pharmaceutical research and development: What do we get for all that money?" *British Medical Journal* 344 (2012): 1–5.

Light, Donald W., Joel R. Lexchin, J., and Jonathan J. Darrow. "Institutional corruption of pharmaceuticals and the myth of safe and effective drugs," *Journal of Law, Medicine & Ethics* 41, no. 3 (2013): 590–600.

Lipsitz, George. "The meaning of memory: Family, class, and ethnicity in early network television." In *Gender, Race, and Class in Media: A Text Reader.* 2nd edition, edited by Gail Dines and Jean M. Humez, 40–47. Thousand Oaks: Sage, 2003.

Long, John C. "Foucault's clinic," *The Journal of Medical Humanities* 13, no. 3 (1992): 119–138, doi: 10.1007/BF01127371.

Lyles, Alan. "Direct marketing of pharmaceuticals to consumers," *Annual Review of Public Health* 23 (2002): 73–91.

MacRury, Iain. *Advertising: Routledge Introductions to Media and Communications.* London: Routledge, 2009.

Main, Kelley J., Jennifer J. Argo, and Bruce A. Huhmann. "Pharmaceutical advertising in the USA: Information or influence?" *International Journal of Advertising* 23 (2004): 119–142.

Manganello, Jennifer, and Martin Fishbein. "Using theory to inform content analysis." In *Media Messages and Public Health: A Decisions Approach to Content Analysis*, edited by Dale J. Kunkel, Jennifer Manganello, and Martin Fishbein, 3–14. New York: Taylor & Francis, 2009.

Marcia, Angell. "Excess in the pharmaceutical industry," *Canadian Medical Association* 171, no. 12 (2004): 1451–1453, doi: 10.1503/cmaj.1041594.

Marshall, Barbara L. "Sexual medicine, sexual bodies and 'pharmaceutical imagination'," *Science as Culture* 18 (2009): 133–149, doi: 10.1080/09505430902885466.

Martin, Emily. "The pharmaceutical person," *BioSocieties* 1 (2006): 273–287, doi: 10.1017/S1745855206003012.

Marx, Karl. *Capital: Volume 1: A Critique of Political Economy*. Translated by Ben Fowkes. London: Penguin Books, 1992.

Mastin, Teresa, Julie L. Andsager, Jounghwa Choi, and Kyungjin Lee. "Health disparities anddirect-to-consumer prescription drug advertising: A content analysis of targeted magazine genres, 1992–2002," *Health Communication* 22 (2007): 49–58, doi: 10.1080/10410230701310299.

McAllister, Matthew P., and Emily West. *The Routledge Companion to Advertising and Promotional Culture*. New York: Routledge, 2013.

McAllister, Matthew P. "Commodity fetishism." In *Encyclopedia of Consumption and Consumer Studies*, edited by Daniel Thomas Cook and J. Michael Ryan. Hoboken: Wiley-Blackwell, 2014.

McAllister, Matthew P. "AIDS, Medicalization, and the News Media." In *AIDS: A Communication Perspective*, edited by Timthy Edgar, Mary Anne Fitzpatrick, and Vicki S. Freimuth, 195–221. Hillsdale: Lawrence Erlbaum, 1992.

McCaffrey, Kevin. "OTC Nexium launches amid generic uncertainty," *Medical Marketing & Media*, May 27, 2014. http://www.mmm-online.com/otc-nexium-launches-amid-generic-uncertainty/article/348664/.

Meehan, Eileen R. "Gendering the commodity audience: Critical media research, feminism, and political economy." In *Sex and Money: Feminism and Political Economy in the Media*, edited by Eileen R. Meehan and Ellen Riordan, 209–222. Minneapolis: University of Minnesota Press, 2002.

Meghani, Zahra, and Jennifer Kuzma. "The 'revolving door' between regulatory agencies and industry: A problem that requires reconceptualizing objectivity," *Journal of Agricultural and Environmental Ethics* 24, no. 6 (2011): 575–599, doi: 10.1007/s10806-010-9287-x.

Merck. "Basic Training Participant Guide," 2002. http://oversight.house.gov/features/vioxx/documents.asp.

Merck. "Nasonex," CBS, Television advertisement, aired 15 April 2010.

Meyer, Richard. "Majority of physicians believe DTC ads should be cut back," April 30, 2013. http://www.worldofdtcmarketing.com.

Mintzes, Barbara. "For and against: Direct to consumer advertising is medicalising normal human experience," *British Medical Journal* 324, no. 7342 (2002): 908–909.

Morgan, Steven G., Kenneth L. Bassett, James M. Wright, Robert G. Evans, Morris L. Barer, Patricia A. Caetano, and Charlyn D. Black. "'Breakthrough' drugs and growth in expenditure on prescription drugs in Canada," *British Medical Journal* 331 (2005): 815–816, doi: 10.1136/bmj.38582.703866.AE.

Motola, Domeico, Fabrizio De Ponti, Elisabetta Poluzzi, Nelb Martini, Pasqualino Rossi, Maria Chiara Silvani, Alberto Vaccheri, and Nicola Montanaro. "An update on the first decadeof the European centralized procedure: How many innovative drugs?" *British Journal of Clinical Pharmacology* 62 (2006): 610–616, doi: 10.1111/j.1365-2125.2006.02700.x.

Moynihan, Ray, and David Henry. "The fight against disease mongering: Generating knowledge for action," *PLoS Medicine* 3, no. 4 (2006): 425–428, doi: 10.1371/journal.pmed.0030191.

Nathanson, Constance A. *Dangerous Passage: The Social Control of Sexuality in Women's Adolescence*. Philadelphia: Temple University Press, 1991.

Neuendorf, Kimberly A. *The Content Analysis Guidebook*. Thousand Oaks: Sage, 2002.

Neuhaus, Jessamyn. *Housework and Housewives in American Advertising: Married to the Mop*. New York: Palgrave Macmillan, 2011.

Nussbaum, Jon F. *Intergenerational Communication across the Lifespan*. Mahwah: Lawrence Erlbaum, 2001.

O'Barr, William. *Culture and the Ad: Exploring Otherness in the World of Advertising*. Boulder: Westview Press, 1994.

Palmer, Eric, and Carly Helfand. "The Top 10 Pharma Companies by 2013 Revenue," 2014. http://www.fiercepharma.com/special-reports/top-10-pharma-companies-2013-revenue.

Palumbo, Francis B., and C. Daniel Mullins. "The development of direct-to-consumer prescription drug advertising regulation," *Food and Drug Law Journal* 57, no. 3 (2002).

Parsons, Patricia J. "Integrating ethics with strategy: Analyzing disease-branding," *Corporate Communications: An International Journal* 12, no. 3 (2007): 267–279. doi: http://dx.doi.org/10.1108/13563280710776860.

Payer, Lynn. *Disease-Mongers: How Doctors, Drug Companies and Insurers Are Making You Feel Sick*. New York: Wiley, 1992.

Pearce, Kevin, and Stanley Baran. "Still critical after all these years? Direct-to-Consumer prescription drug advertising as object lesson," Paper presented at the Annual Meeting for the National Communication Association, November 2008.

Peerson, Anita. "Foucault and modern medicine," *Nursing Inquiry* 2 (1995): 106–114, doi: 10.1111/j.1440-1800.1995.tb00073.x.

Pfizer. "Lyrica Version One," ABC. Television advertisement, aired 2 April 2010a.

Pfizer. "Lyrica Version Two," CBS. Television advertisement, aired 7 February 2010b.

Pfizer. "Lipitor Version One," CBS. Television advertisement, aired 1 April 2010c.

Pfizer. "Viagra," CBS. Television advertisement, aired 14 April 2010d.

Phillipov, Michelle. "In defense of textual analysis: Resisting methodological hegemony in media and cultural studies," *Critical Studies in Media Communication* 30, no. 3 (2013): 209–223, doi: 10.1080/15295036.2011.639380.

Post, Ashley. "Bayer accused of promoting Yaz birth control for unapproved uses," *InsideCounsel*, November 21, 2011.

"Prescription Drug Trends," *The Henry J. Kaiser Family Foundation*, May 2007, http://www.kff.org/rxdrugs/upload/3057_06.pdf.

Pulvirenti, Mariastella, John McMillan, and Sharon Lawn. "Empowerment, patient centered care and self-management," *Health Expectations* 17, no. 3 (2011): 303–310, doi: 10.1111/j.1369-7625.2011.00757.x.

Quesinberry Stokes, Ashli. "Health literacy in DTCA 2.0: Digital and social media frontiers." In *The Routledge Companion to Advertising and Promotional Culture*, edited by Matthew P. McAllister and Emily West, 285–297. New York: Routledge, 2013.

Rhee, James. "The influence of the pharmaceutical industry on healthcare practitioners' prescribing habits," *The Internet Journal of Academic Physician Assistants* 7 (2008).

Richter, S. "The real bayer fallout," *Chief Executive*, February 2002.

Riffe, Daniel, Stephen Lacy, and Frederick G. Fico. *Analyzing Media Messages: Using Quantitative Content Analysis in Research*. 2nd edition. Mahwah: Lawrence Erlbaum, 2005.

Riordan, Ellen. "Commodified agent and empowered girls: Consuming and producing feminism," *Journal of Communication Inquiry* 25, no. 3 (2001): 279-297, doi: 10.1177/0196859901025003006.

Roche Group. "Boniva," ABC. Television advertisement, aired 10 February 2010.

Rose, Nikolas. "Beyond medicalization," *Lancet* 369 (2007): 700–702.

Rosenberg, Charles E. "The tyranny of diagnosis: Specific entities and individual experience," *Milbank Quarterly* 80, no. 2 (2002): 237, doi: 10.1111/1468-0009. t01-1-00003.

Rosenfield, Dana, and Christopher A. Faircloth. *Medicalized Masculinities*. Philadelphia: Temple University Press, 2006.

Rosenthal, Meredith B., Ernst R. Berndt, Julie M. Donohue, Arnold M. Epstein, and Richard G. Frank. "Demand effects of recent changes in prescription drug promotion," *The Henry J. Kaiser Family Foundation*, June 2003, http://www.kff.org/rxdrugs/6084-index.cfm.

Schiller, Herbert I. *Mass Communication and American Empire*, 2nd edition. Boulder: Westview Press, 1992.

Schooler, Caroline, Michael D. Basil, and David G. Altman. "Alcohol and cigarette advertising and billboards: Targeting with social cues," *Health Communication* 8 (1996): 109–129.

Shuchman, Miriam, and Michael S. Wilkes. "The vitamin uprising," *New York Times Magazine*, October 2 (1994): 79.

Scitovsky, Tibor. *Welfare and Competition*. Revised edition. Chicago: Richard D. Irwin, 1971.

Sender, Katherine. "Selling sexual subjectivities: Audiences respond to gay window advertising," *Critical Studies in Media Communication* 16 (1999): 172–196.

Siegel Watkins, Elizabeth. "How the pill became a lifestyle drug: The pharmaceutical industry and birth control in the United States since 1960," *Public Health Then and Now* 102, no. 8 (2012): 1462–1472, doi: 10.2105/AJPH.2012.300706.

Silverman, David. *Interpreting Qualitative Data: Methods for Analyzing Talk, Text and Interaction.* 3rd edition. London: Sage, 2006.

Smythe, Dallas W. *Communications, Capitalism, Consciousness, and Canada.* Norwood: Ablex, 1980.

Spigel, Lynn. *Make Room for TV: Television and the Family Ideal in Postwar America.* Chicago: University of Chicago Press, 1992.

Spigel, Lynn. "Designing the smart house: Posthuman domesticity and conspicuous production," *European Journal of Cultural Studies* 8, no. 4 (2005): 403–426, doi: 10.1177/1367549405057826.

Steinbrook, Robert. "For sale: Physicians' prescribing data," *The New England Journal of Medicine* 354 (2006): 2745–2747.

Steinem, Gloria. "Sex, lies and advertising." In *Gender, Race, and Class in Media: A Text Reader.* 2nd edition, edited by Gail Dines and Jean M. Humez, 223–229. Thousand Oaks: Sage, 2003.

Stole, Inger L. "The fight against critics and the discovery of 'Spin': American advertising in the 1930s and 1940s." In *The Routledge Companion to Advertising and Promotional Culture*, edited by Matthew P. McAllister and Emily West, 39–52. New York: Routledge, 2013.

Strasser, Susan. *Satisfaction Guaranteed: The Making of the Mass Market.* New York: Pantheon Books, 1989.

Strasser, Susan. "The alien past: Consumer culture in historical perspective." In *The Advertising and Consumer Culture Reader*, edited by Joseph Turow and Matthew P. McAllister, 25–37. New York: Routledge, 2009.

Stein, Sarah R. "The '1984' Macintosh ad: Cinematic icons and constitutive rhetoric in the launch of a new machine," *Quarterly Journal of Speech* 88, no. 2 (2002): 169–192.

Stephens, Nancy. "Cognitive age: A useful concept for advertising?" *Journal of Advertising* 20, no. 4 (1991): 37–48.

Symm, Barbalee, Michael Averitt, Samuel N. Forjuoh, and Cheryl Preece. "Effects of using free sample medications on the prescribing practices of family physicians," *Journal of the American Board of Family Medicine* 19, no. 5 (2006): 443–449, doi: 10.3122/jabfm.19.5.443.

Taylor, Timothy D. "Music in the new capitalism." In *The International Encyclopedia of Media Studies: Vol. 2: Media Production*, edited by Angharad N. Valdivia, 151–170. Oxford: Wiley-Blackwell, 2013.

The Federal Food, Drug, and Cosmetic Act, 52 U.S. Stat. (1938), § 1040.

The Pure Food and Drugs Act, 34 U.S. Stat. (1906), § 768.

Thomas, David R. "A general inductive approach for analyzing qualitative evaluation data," *American Journal of Evaluation* 27, no. 2 (2006): 237–246, doi: 10.1177/1098214005283748.

Thompson, Teresa L., Alicia Dorsey, Katherine Miller, and Roxanne Parrott. *Handbook of Health Communication.* Mahwah: Lawrence Erlbaum Associates, 2003.

Tinsley, Howard A., and David J. Weiss. "Interrater reliability and agreement of subjective judgments," *Journal of Counseling Psychology* 22 (1975): 358–376.

"Top 200 Drugs for 2009 by Units Sold," 2010a. http://www.drugs.com/top200_units.html.

"Top 200 Drugs for 2009 by Sales," 2010b. http://www.drugs.com/top200.html.

Tone, Andrea. "Medicalizing reproduction: The pill and home pregnancy tests," *Journal of Sex Research* 49, no. 4 (2012): 319–327, doi: 10.1080/00224499.2012.688226.

Turow, Joseph, and Matthew P. McAllister. *The Advertising and Consumer Culture Reader*. New York: Taylor & Francis, 2009.

U.S. Department of Health. National Center for Health Statistics. *Health, United States, 2013: With Special Feature of Prescription Drugs*. Washington: United States Government Printing Office, 2014.

United States Government Accountability Office. *FDA Oversight of DTC Advertising has Limitations*. GAO-03-177. Washington: United States Government Accountability Office, 2002.

United States Government Accountability Office. *Prescription Drugs: Improvements Needed in FDA's Oversight of Direct-to-Consumer*. Washington: United States Government Accountability Office, 2006.

United States Kefauver Harris Amendment, 21 U.S.C. 301 (1962).

U.S. Office on Women's Health. Department of Health and Human Services. "Premenstrual Syndrome (PMS) Fact Sheet," http://www.womenshealth.gov/publications/our-publications/fact-sheet/premenstrual-syndrome.html#c. 2012.

U.S. Food and Drug Administration Center for Drug Evaluation and Research. Department of Health and Human Services. "NDAs approved in calendar years 1990–2003 by therapeutic potentials and chemical types," www.fda.gov/cder/rdmt/pstable.htm. 2004.

U.S. Food and Drug Administration. Division of Drug Marketing, Advertising, and Communications. "YAZ NDA 21-676/21-873/22-045 Warning Letter," http://www.fda.gov/iceci/enforcementactions/WarningLetters/default.htm. 2008.

U.S. Food and Drug Administration. Division of Drug Marketing, Advertising, and Communications. "YAZ NDA 21-676/21-873/22-045 Warning Letter," http://www.fda.gov/iceci/enforcementactions/WarningLetters/default.htm. 2009.

U.S. Senate. "Lobbying Disclosure Act Database," 2014. http://soprweb.senate.gov/index.cfm?event=selectfields.

van Luijn, Johan C. F., Frank W. Gribnau, and Hubert G. M. Leufkens. "Superior efficacy of new medicines?" *European Journal of Clinical Pharmacology* 66 (2010): 445–448, doi: 10.1007/s00228-010-0808-3.

Ventola, C. Lee. "Direct-to-Consumer pharmaceutical advertising: Therapeutic or toxic?" 2011. http://www.ncbi.nlm.nih.gov.

Vincent, William R. "'Free' prescription drug samples are not free," *American Journal of Public Health* 98, no. 8 (2008): 1348–1359, doi: http://dx.doi.org/10.2105/AJPH.2008.138800.

Wallis, Laura. "Beyond politics: New medical concerns for contraceptive users," *American Journal of Nursing* 112, no. 7 (2012): 19, doi: 10.1097/01.NAJ.0000415945.79418.ef.

Welch Cline, W. M. "Tauzin switches sides from drug industry overseer to lobbyist." USA Today. Retrieved from http://usatoday30.usatoday.com/money/industries/health/drugs/2004-12-15-drugs-usat_x.htm, 2004, December 16

Welch Cline, Rebecca J., and Henry N. Young. "Marketing drugs, marketing health care relationships: A content analysis of visual cues in direct-to-consumer prescription drug advertising," *Health Communication* 16, no. 2 (2004): 131–157.

Weissman, Joel S., Alvin J. Silk, Kinga Zapert, Michael Newman, Robert Leitman, and Sandra Feibelmann. "Physicians report on patient encounters involving direct-to-consumer advertising," *Health Affairs* 10, no. 1377 (2004): W4–219–233.

Wilkes, Michael S., Robert A. Bell, and Richard L. Kravitz. "Direct to consumer prescription drug advertising: trends, impact, and implications," *Health Affairs* 19, no. 2 (2000).

Williams, Raymond. *Materialism and Culture*. London: Verso, 1980.

Williams, Simon J., Jonathan Gabe, and Peter Davis. "The sociology of pharmaceuticals: Progress and prospects," *Sociology of Health & Illness* 30, no. 6 (2008): 813–824, doi: 10.1111/j.1467-9566.2008.01123.x.

Williams, Simon J., Clive Seale, Sharon Boden, Pam Lowe, and Deborah Lynn. "Waking up to sleepiness." In *Pharmaceuticals and Society*, edited by Simon J. Williams, Jonathan Gabe, and Peter Davis, 1–11. Chichester: Wiley-Blackwell, 2009.

Williamson, Judith. *Decoding Advertisements: Ideology and Meaning in Advertising*. London: Marion Boyars, 1978.

Woods, Carly S. "Repunctuated feminism: Marketing menstrual suppression through the rhetoric of choice," *Women's Studies in Communication* 36 (2013): 267–287, doi: 10.1080/07491409.2013.829791.

Yang, Mo, Jeongeun So, Ankur Patel, and Sujit S. Sansgiry. "Content analysis of the videos featuring prescription drug advertisements in social media: YouTube," *Drug Information Journal* 46, no. 6 (2012): 715–722. "YAZ Approval History," 2014. http://www.drugs.com/history/Yaz.html.

Young, James Harvey. *The Medical Messiahs: A Social History of Health Quackery in Twentieth-Century America*. Princeton: Princeton University Press, 1969.

Zubow Poe, Pamela. "Direct-to-consumer drug advertising and 'health media filters': A qualitative study of older adult women's responses to DTC ads," *Atlantic Journal of Communication* 20, no. 3 (2012): 185–199.

Index

About the Author

Dr. Applequist earned her Ph.D. in Mass Communication from the Pennsylvania State University in 2015. She taught and researched at Penn State (where she also received her B.A. and M.A. degrees) prior to joining the faculty at University of South Florida in The Zimmerman School of Advertising and Mass Communication. As a researcher focused on health communication and advertising, Dr. Applequist is interested in the pharmaceutical industry, especially in regards to developing more normative frameworks to encourage proper patient education. She has presented her research at a number of conferences, including forums abroad in Australia and Italy. Her research explores the content of pharmaceutical advertisements, legal compliance with Food and Drug Administration (FDA) requirements, and issues of representation related to patients and health care in these advertisements. Dr. Applequist is especially passionate about her teaching and had the privilege to convey that message in her TEDx talk in 2014. She is currently an undergraduate and graduate faculty member, teaching *Qualitative Research Methods in Mass Communications* at the graduate level, and *Principles of Public Relations, Health Communication and the Media*, and *Media and the 2016 Election* at the undergraduate level.